SELF-ASSESSMENT in HUMAN ANATOMY

Assisted by

Prof Baitullah
BSc (Hons), MBBS, MS

Prof S.J. Haider
MBBS, MS, FRMS (England)

Dr Mobarak Hossain
MBBS, MD

Dr Aijaz A. Khan
MBBS, MS, Ph.D

Dr Farah Ghaus
MBBS, MS

Dr Mohammad Aslam
MBBS, DLO, MS

SELF-ASSESSMENT in HUMAN ANATOMY

for
☐ Quick Revision ☐ Self-Assessment and
☐ Postgraduate Medical Entrance Examination

Nafis Ahmad Faruqi
MBBS, MS, MNYAS (USA), Man of Y2K2 (USA)

Professor, Department of Anatomy
Jawaharlal Nehru Medical College,
Aligarh Muslim University
Aligarh 202002, India

Arsalan Moinuddin
MBBS

Gulfishan, Allahwali Kothi,
Dodhpur, Civil Lines
Aligarh 202002, India

CBS
CBS Publishers and Distributors Pvt Ltd
New Delhi • Bangalore • Pune • Cochin • Chennai

SELF-ASSESSMENT in HUMAN ANATOMY

ISBN: 978-81-239-1784-9

First Edition: 2010

Published by Satish Kumar Jain and produced by Vinod K. Jain for
CBS Publishers & Distributors Pvt Ltd
4819/XI Prahlad Street, 24 Ansari Road, Daryaganj,
New Delhi 110 002, India.   Website: www.cbspd.com
Ph: 23289259, 23266861, 23266867   Fax: 011-23243014   e-mail: delhi@cbspd.com

Branches

* Bangalore: Seema House 2975, 17th Cross, K.R. Road,
  Banasankari 2nd Stage, Bangalore 560 070, Karnataka
  Ph: 26771678/79   Fax: 080-26771680   e-mail: cbsbng@gmail.com
* Pune: Shaan Brahmha Complex, 631/632 Basement,
  Appa Balwant Chowk, Budhwar Peth, next to Ratan Talkies,
  Pune 411 002, Maharashtra
  Ph: 020-24464057/58   Fax: 020-24464059   e-mail: pune@cbspd.com
* Cochin: 36/14 Kalluvilakam, Lissie Hospital Road,
  Cochin 682 018, Kerala
  Ph: 0484-4059061-65   Fax: 0484-4059065   e-mail: cochin@cbspd.com
* Chennai: 20, West Park Road, Shenoy Nagar, Chennai 600 030, TN
  Ph: 044-26260666, 26202620   Fax: 044-45530020   email: chennai@cbspd.com

Typeset at Limited Colors, Delhi 110 092
Printed at Somya Printers, Delhi-110 053

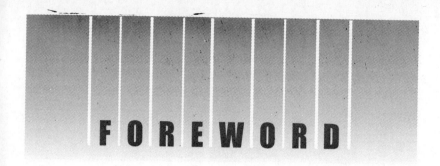

FOREWORD

I feel greatly privileged in writing the Foreword to the book *Self-Assessment in Human Anatomy* by Dr Nafis Ahmad Faruqi and Dr Arsalan Moinuddin.

The authors have worked hard in preparation of the manuscript and I am confident that for the students of anatomy this book is ideal for self-assessment and rapid revision.

Dr Muzammil Ullah
Ex-Professor, Department of Anatomy
Jawaharlal Nehru Medical College
Aligarh Muslim University, Aligarh

PREFACE

The present work entitled *Self-Assessment in Human Anatomy* is primarily meant to help the medical students to evaluate their own knowledge in the subject of human anatomy. It differs from the traditional MCQs books as it also provides a wealth of relevant information on the subject including its applied aspects. The simplicity and clarity in expression has been taken into account throughout. A special feature of this book is the additional key with correct statements which has made it more useful to its readers.

We are highly grateful to Prof A Halim and Prof DN Sinha who have been kind enough to go through the manuscript and give their expert opinions and suggestions.

Nafis Ahmad Faruqi
Arsalan Moinuddin

CONTENTS

CONTENTS

UPPER LIMB

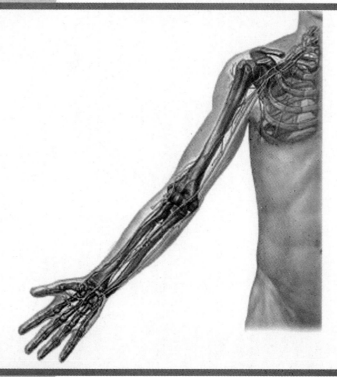

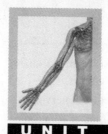

UPPER LIMB

Find out incorrect statement in each set.

1. Clavicle

(a) It is the only long bone lying horizontally.
(b) It has no medullary cavity.
(c) It is second to mandible to ossify.
(d) Intermediate supraclavicular nerve may pierce it.
(e) It is fractured most commonly at junction of its two curvatures.

2. Jugular notch

(a) It is present at upper end of manubrium sterni.
(b) Investing layer of cervical fascia splits and gets attached to its anterior and posterior margins to enclose space of Burns.
(c) Jugular arch connecting the two external jugular veins, lies above the jugular notch.
(d) Fibres of interclavicular ligament are fused with jugular notch.
(e) Sternal (tendinous) head of sternocleidomastoid is attached to it.

3. Pectoral region

(a) Skin above the level of angle of Louis is supplied by cutaneous branches of 1st intercostal nerve.

3

(b) As the adjacent dermatomes overlap considerably, a single segment lesion may fail to cause any anaesthesia.

(e) Pectoralis major is supplied by both the pectoral nerves.

(d) Pectoralis minor assists in protraction and medial rotation of scapula.

(e) Most of lymphatics of the region drain into axillary lymph nodes.

4. The breast

(a) Mammary ridge extends from axilla to inguinal region.

(b) Vertically, breast extends from 2nd to 6th ribs in midclavicular line.

(c) Radial incision in breast is preferred to prevent mammary glands from damage.

(d) Incision along inferior margin of breast is the most suitable, from cosmetic view point.

(e) Most of lymphatics from breast drain into internal mammary group of lymph nodes.

5. Clavipectoral fascia

(a) It strengthens posterior wall of axilla.

(b) It splits to enclose pectoralis minor and subclavius.

(c) It extends from clavicle to axillary fascia.

(d) Its thickened part between 1st rib and coracoid process is named as costocoracoid ligament.

(e) It is pierced by cephalic vein, thoracoacromial artery, lateral pectoral nerve and lymphatics.

6. Axilla

(a) Its medial wall is wider than its lateral wall.

(b) Apex of axilla is triangular in shape.

(c) Deep fascia in the floor of axilla is called axillary fascia.

(d) Axillary arch is an occasional muscular slip extending between latissimus dorsi and pectoralis major.

(e) Axillary tail (of Spence) of breast pierces the anterior wall to enter axilla.

7. Axillary vessels

(a) Subclavian artery continues as axillary artery beyond outer border of 1st rib.

(b) The relations of cords of brachial plexus to 1st part of axillary artery are indicated by their names.

(c) Lateral thoracic artery, a branch of 2nd part of axillary artery, is a significant source of blood supply for female breast.

(d) Basilic vein continues as axillary vein at lower border of teres major.

(e) Axillary artery together with brachial plexus is enclosed in axillary sheath, derived from prevertebral lamina of cervical fascia.

8. Brachial plexus

(a) Cords of brachial plexus lie behind the clavicle.

(b) Difficult child birth may result into Erb-Duchenne paralysis (adduction of arm and pronation of forearm, called "porter's tip" deformity).

(c) Branches from the cords of brachial plexus arise below the lower border of pectoralis minor.

(d) Klumpke's paralysis, caused by violent hyperabduction of arm, leads to "claw hand" deformity.

(e) Prefixed brachial plexus receives an additional root from 4th cervical ventral ramus.

9. Cutaneous nerves of back

(a) Obliquity of descent of cutaneous branches of dorsal rami makes the thoracic dermatomes almost horizontal.

(b) In upper part of body, lateral branches, while in lower part, medial branches of dorsal rami give rise to cutaneous twigs.

(c) The integrity of dorsal rami failing to reach skin cannot be assured by testing the corresponding dermatomes.

(d) In addition to sensory fibres to skin, cutaneous branches also carry the sympathetic fibres to arrector pili, sweat glands and blood vessels.

(e) No cutaneous branches are given off by dorsal rami of the 1st and the last two cervical and the last two lumbar nerves.

10. Trapezius

(a) Its upper fibres along with levator scapulae elevate the scapula.

(b) Its lower fibres converge to form a tendon to be inserted on the erroneously named deltoid tubercle of scapular spine.

(c) Both its sensory and motor supply are derived from accessory spinal nerve.

(d) Its middle fibres help in retraction of scapula.

(e) Its upper and lower fibres together assist the serratus anterior in lateral rotation of scapula, during abduction of arm above head.

11. Scapula

(a) Elevation of its medial border (winging of scapula) results from paralysis of the serratus anterior.

(b) Fracture of scapula is uncommon due to the cushion provided by scapular muscles.

(c) It extends vertically from 2nd to 7th ribs.

(d) The centre of ossification appearing during 1st year in middle of coracoid process is an example of atavistic epiphysis.

(e) Long heads of biceps brachii and triceps arise from infraglenoid and supraglenoid tubercles, respectively.

12. Movements of scapula

(a) Serratus anterior is the most powerful protractor.

(b) Scapular rotation contributes about one-third (60°) in 180° abduction.

(c) Protraction and retraction take place between articular disc and lateral end of clavicle at acromioclavicular joint.

(d) Most important stabilizing factor during scapular movements at acromioclavicular joint is coracoacromial ligament.

(e) Rhomboids are principally retractors of scapula.

13. Latissimus dorsi

(a) It is covered by trapezius.

(b) It is the only muscle in body connecting lower limb with upper limb.

(c) Its innervation is derived from long thoracic nerve (of Bell).

(d) A branch of subscapular artery, called thoracodorsal artery, supplies the latissimus dorsi.

(e) It is adductor, extensor and medial rotator of the arm.

14. Humerus

(a) Its upper end is the growing end.

(b) The nutrient canal is directed downwards.

(c) Surgical neck is the narrow junction of its upper end and shaft.

(d) The common epiphysis at its lower end is the first, of all long bone epiphyses, to fuse with the shaft.

(e) Back of its lateral epicondyle provides attachment to common extensor origin.

15. Radius

(a) Thrust on hand is transmitted through its lower end.

(b) Its lower end is the growing end.

(c) The nutrient canal is directed upwards.

(d) Colles' fracture involves its upper end.

(e) Due to possible injury to posterior interosseous nerve, the exposure of the radius is avoided from back.

16. Ulna

(a) Its posterior border is covered with muscles.

(b) The ossification centre for its upper end appears later than the centre for its lower end.

(c) Fracture of olecranon is difficult to manage due to strong pull of the triceps.

(d) Its surgical exposure is preferably done from back.

(e) The ulnar styloid process lies at a higher level and more posteriorly than the styloid process of radius.

17. Carpal bones

(a) Scaphoid is the commonest to fracture.

(b) Swelling and tenderness in anatomical snuff-box indicate fracture of lunate.

(c) Carpal bones are arranged in such a way that they together produce a concavity on the palmar aspect, through which pass the flexor tendons.

(d) Trapezium forms a saddle type of synovial joint with base of 1st metacarpal.

(e) The commonest carpal bone to be dislocated is lunate.

18. Superficial veins of upper limb

(a) Basilic vein runs along postaxial (ulnar) border of upper limb.

(b) Median cubital vein is the vein of choice for intravenous injections.

(c) Cephalic vein drains into subclavian vein.

(d) Bicipital aponeurosis separates median cubital vein, lying superficial to it, from median nerve and brachial artery, located deep to it.

(e) Cephalic vein may communicate with external jugular vein via a connecting vein crossing clavicle.

19. Lymphatic drainage of upper limb

(a) Superficial lymphatics accompany the veins.

(b) Lymphatics from pectoral region drain mainly into anterior group of axillary lymph nodes.

(c) Supratrochlear lymph nodes receive lymphatics from the lateral fingers.

   (d) Lymphatics from scapular region drain into posterior group of axillary lymph nodes.

   (e) Secondaries in central group of axillary lymph nodes may lead to referred pain in upper medial arm, due to its intimate relationship with lateral branch of 2nd intercostal (intercostobrachial) nerve.

20. Cutaneous nerves of upper limb

   (a) In brachial block, anaesthesia is incomplete in the axillary floor.

   (b) Skin over upper part of deltoid is supplied by lateral supraclavicular nerve.

   (c) The dorsal aspects of distal parts of lateral three and half digits are innervated by the radial nerve.

   (d) Posterior cutaneous nerve of forearm arises from the radial nerve.

   (e) Medial cutaneous nerve of forearm also supplies medial aspect of lower arm, in addition to that of forearm.

21. Dermatomes of upper limb

   (a) Area of skin supplied by single spinal nerve is called dermatome.

   (b) There is little overlapping between continuous adjacent dermatomes.

   (c) Axial lines demarcate junctions of discontinuous segments.

   (d) Anterior axial line extends from angle of Louis to front of lower forearm.

   (e) Posterior axial line stretches between vertebra prominens and back of elbow.

22. Deep fascia of upper limb

   (a) Biceps brachii, in addition to its insertion on the radial tuberosity, is also attached to the ulna through deep fascia of forearm.

   (b) Medial and lateral intermuscular septa of the arm are well defined only in its lower half.

(c) Deep fascia of forearm is firmly fixed to posterior border of radius.

(d) Deep fascia does not pass freely over subcutaneous parts of the bones.

(e) Flexor retinaculum is thickened deep fascia attached to the four marginal carpal bones.

23. Deltoid

(a) Its acromial part consists of large parallel fibres.

(b) Deltoid paralysis may result from the fracture of humerus at its surgical neck.

(c) It is the main abductor of arm.

(d) Its clavicular fibres flex and medially rotate the arm.

(e) Its innervation is derived from axillary (circumflex) nerve.

24. Supraspinatus

(a) It is the main muscle to initiate abduction of arm.

(b) Subacromial bursa lies between it and acromion process.

(c) Rupture of supraspinatus tendon may lead to a communication between subacromial bursa and cavity of shoulder joint.

(d) It is attached on top of greater tubercle of humerus.

(e) It is innervated by upper subscapular branch of posterior cord.

25. Acromioclavicular joint

(a) The articular disc, often present inside the joint, is usually a complete one.

(b) Both of its articular surfaces slope downwards and medially.

(c) Its principal stabilizing factor is coracoclavicular ligament.

(d) During its dislocation, the clavicle overrides the acromion.

(e) It is a plane type of synovial joint.

26. Shoulder joint

(a) It is a very unstable ball and socket type of synovial joint.

(b) Its ligaments form the most important stabilizing factor.

(c) Of the large joints, it is the commonest to dislocate.

(d) Head of the humerus faces medially, upwards and backwards.

(e) The abduction at glenohumeral joint may be as high as 120°.

27. Axillary nerve

(a) It passes through quadrangular muscular space along with posterior circumflex humeral artery.

(b) It arises from posterior cord of brachial plexus.

(c) It supplies the muscles (deltoid and teres minor) only.

(d) It may be injured in fracture of humerus at its surgical neck.

(e) It carries fibres from 5th and 6th cervical spinal segments.

28. Anastomoses around scapula

(a) The branches from subclavian and axillary arteries participate in these anastomoses.

(b) Suprascapular artery passes above the transverse (superior) scapular ligament.

(c) Dorsal scapular neurovascular bundle runs along the medial border of scapula.

(d) These anastomoses provide collateral circulation, when there is obstruction between origins of thyrocervical trunk and subscapular artery.

(e) Circumflex scapular artery is a branch of suprascapular artery.

29. Biceps brachii

(a) The tendon of its long head, attached to supraglenoid tubercle, is intracapsular.

(b) Its short head and coracobrachialis have got a common attachment to tip of coracoid process.

(c) It is a flexor at elbow and a powerful supinator of flexed forearm.

(d) It is one of the muscles involved in Klumpke's paralysis.

(e) Its tendon of insertion is attached to the posterior aspect of radial tuberosity.

30. Cubital fossa

(a) It is bounded medially by pronator teres, and laterally by brachioradialis.

(b) Supinator and brachialis lie in its floor.

(c) In the fossa, median nerve is sandwiched between brachial artery and tendon of biceps brachii.

(d) Bicipital aponeurosis descends medially to fuse with deep fascia of forearm.

(e) Brachial artery usually terminates in the fossa at level of neck of radius.

31. Musculocutaneous nerve

(a) It arises from lateral cord of brachial plexus.

(b) It passes downwards and lateralwards through the coracobrachialis.

(c) After supplying muscles of flexor compartment of arm, it continues as medial cutaneous nerve of forearm.

(d) It gives off an articular twig to the elbow joint.

(e) It receives nerve fibres from cervical spinal segments 5, 6, 7.

32. Ulnar nerve

(a) Its root value is cervical 7, 8 and thoracic 1 spinal segments.

(b) In the axilla, it lies in between the axillary vessels.

(c) In lower half of arm, it accompanies superior ulnar collateral branch of brachial artery.

(d) It is directly related to back of medial epicondyle of humerus.

(e) It gives off, number of branches to muscles of the arm.

33. Median nerve in arm

(a) It is formed, by the union of its medial and lateral roots, on the medial aspect of 3rd part of the axillary artery.

(b) No muscular branch arises from it in the arm.

(c) It runs first on the lateral side of the brachial artery, and then after crossing it in front, descends on its medial aspect.

(d) It passes deep to bicipital aponeurosis.

(e) It may be involved during ligation of the brachial artery.

34. Brachial artery

(a) It is the continuation of axillary artery beyond lower margin of teres major.

(b) It can be easily palpated in middle of arm against humerus.

(c) It terminates at level of neck of radius by dividing into anterior and posterior interosseous arteries.

(d) Profunda brachii is usually the highest branch arising from it.

(e) It is accompanied by venae comitantes, also called brachial veins.

35. Triceps

(a) It has three heads of origin-long, lateral and medial.

(b) Tendon of triceps gets attached to posterior part of superior surface of olecranon process of ulna.

(c) Its long head supports the shoulder joint from below during abduction of arm.

(d) All its three heads are innervated by a single branch of the radial nerve.

(e) Articularis cubiti (subanconeus) consists of few fibres of its medial head attached to posterior aspect of capsule of elbow joint.

36. Radial nerve in arm

(a) Its root value is cervical 5, 6, 7, 8 and thoracic 1 spinal segments.

(b) It is commonly injured in midhumeral shaft fracture.

(c) It courses only in extensor compartment of arm.

(d) Radial injury leads to unopposed flexion of hand (wrist drop).

(e) In the radial groove, it is accompanied by profunda brachii artery.

37. Front of forearm

(a) All the flexor compartment muscles of forearm are supplied by median nerve except flexor carpi ulnaris and medial part of flexor digitorum profundus, which are supplied by ulnar nerve.

(b) Flexor digitorum superficialis is the most superficial muscle in front of forearm.

(c) Pronator teres is one of the superficial most, while pronator quadratus is the deepest of flexors of forearm.

(d) Volkmann's ischaemic contracture involves the flexor muscles of forearm.

(e) Superficial branch of radial nerve (radial nerve in forearm) descends between extensor and flexor muscle groups of forearm.

38. Palmar aponeurosis

(a) It is the central thickened deep fascia of palm.

(b) It receives attachment of palmaris longus tendon at its proximal end.

(c) Distally, it divides into five slips, one for each digit.

(d) Dupuytren's contracture usually leads to shortening of medial part of palmar aponeurosis, and consequently flexion of little and ring fingers.

(e) It is firmly adherent to thickened skin of palm.

39. Superficial palmar arch

(a) It is formed by continuation of radial artery in hand.

(b) It is superficial to long flexor tendons, lumbricals and branches of median nerve in hand.

(c) Distally, it extends up to level of distal margin of extended thumb.

(d) Three common palmar digital arteries spring from its convexity towards medial three interdigital clefts.

(e) It lies deep to palmar aponeurosis.

40. Flexor retinaculum

(a) It is attached to four marginal bony prominences—tubercle of scaphoid, crest of trapezium, pisiform and hook of hamate.

(b) Tendon of flexor carpi radialis passes through its lateral part.

(c) Ulnar nerve and ulnar artery enter the palm superficial to it.

(d) Long flexor tendons along with median nerve pass deep to it to enter the hand.

(e) Carpal tunnel syndrome is produced by compression of the structures other than median nerve lying deep to it.

41. Synovial sheaths of flexor tendons

(a) A common synovial sheath (ulnar bursa) encloses tendons of flexor digitorum superficialis and profundus.

(b) The tendons in ulnar bursa invaginate from lateral side.

(c) Radial bursa is the synovial sheath for tendon of flexor carpi radialis.

(d) Tenosynovitis is inflammation of the synovial sheath of a tendon.

(e) Vincula are vascular connective tissue bands on dorsal aspects of flexor tendons of digits.

42. Arteries of flexor compartment of forearm

(a) Radial artery passes superficial to pronator teres along with superficial branch of radial nerve on its lateral aspect.

(b) Ulnar artery descends deep to pronator teres accompanied by ulnar nerve on its medial side.

(c) Anterior interosseous artery and its branches remain confined to flexor compartment of forearm.

(d) Nutrient arteries, both for radius and ulna, spring from anterior interosseous artery.

(e) Radial artery in lower forearm is commonly palpated for pulse observations.

43. Median nerve in forearm and hand

(a) It runs between two heads of pronator teres.

(b) The ulnar artery courses inferomedially deep to median nerve.

(c) Anterior interosseous nerve, a branch of median nerve, supplies all the deep muscles of flexor compartment of forearm except medial part of flexor digitorum profundus.

(d) Median nerve injury in forearm differs from carpal tunnel syndrome, as in the former condition cutaneous sensation over thenar eminence remains intact.

(e) In hand, this nerve supplies muscles of thenar eminence and lateral two lumbricals.

44. Ulnar nerve in forearm and hand

(a) It passes between two heads of flexor carpi ulnaris to enter the forearm.

(b) In forearm, it descends on medial side of ulnar artery.

(c) Its superficial terminal branch is not solely cutaneous, but also innervates the muscle, palmaris brevis.

(d) It supplies all the muscles of hand except muscles of thenar eminence and lateral two lumbricals.

(e) Its injury leads to "claw hand" deformity, in which there is flexion at metacarpophalangeal joints and extension at interphalangeal joints.

45. Fascial compartments of palm

(a) Thenar and midpalmar spaces lie dorsal to common synovial sheath (ulnar bursa) with its long flexor tendons, and lumbricals.

(b) Tenosynovitis in little finger is likely to involve thenar space.

(c) Pus in thenar space can be drained by opening the 1st lumbrical canal.

(d) Midpalmar space suppuration is drained by an incision in 3rd or 4th interdigital cleft.

(e) Involvement of midpalmar space does affect the concavity of the palm.

46. Short muscles of thumb

(a) Thenar eminence is produced by abductor pollicis brevis, flexor pollicis brevis, opponens pollicis and adductor pollicis.

(b) All the short muscles of thumb are supplied by median nerve, except adductor pollicis (always) and flexor pollicis brevis (sometimes), which are supplied by ulnar nerve.

(c) Book test is a reliable clinical test for paralysis of adductor pollicis.

(d) Opponens pollicis brings about movement of 1st metacarpal.

(e) Adduction and abduction of thumb take place in sagittal plane, which is perpendicular to the plane of palm.

47. Short muscles of little finger

(a) Hypothenar eminence consists of only three muscles.

(b) Palmaris brevis is supplied by superficial branch of the ulnar nerve.

(c) Opponens digiti minimi brings about flexion and lateral rotation of 5th metacarpal at carpometacarpal joint.

(d) Flexion of little finger takes place in sagittal palne (at right angle to palmar plane).

(e) Deep branch of ulnar nerve passes between flexor digiti minimi brevis and abductor digiti minimi.

48. Deep palmar arch

(a) It is formed by continuation of radial artery in hand.

(b) It lies at level of proximal margin of extended thumb.

(c) Three common palmar digital arteries arise directly from deep palmar arch.

(d) Deep branch of ulnar nerve lies in concavity of deep palmar arch.

(e) Recurrent branches of deep palmar arch join palmar carpal arch.

49. Extensor compartment of forearm

(a) All the muscles are supplied by deep division of radial nerve except brachioradialis and extensor carpi radialis longus, which are innervated directly by radial nerve.

(b) Deep division of radial nerve (commonly called posterior interosseous nerve) passes between two heads of supinator.

(c) Tendon of extensor pollicis longus grooves the dorsal tubercle (of Lister) of radius on its lateral aspect.

(d) Anconeus is supposedly a detached part of triceps as it is supplied by the nerve to medial head of triceps.

(e) Brachioradialis is a flexor of midpronated forearm.

50. Extensor retinaculum

(a) It is an oblique thickened band of deep fascia attached laterally, to anterior border of radius and medially, to triquetral and pisiform.

(b) Five septa are given off from its deeper aspect to form six compartments.

(c) The most lateral compartment is traversed by tendons of abductor pollicis longus and extensor pollicis brevis.

(d) Branches of superficial division of radial nerve pass superficial to the retinaculum to supply the skin.

(e) Tendon of extensor digiti minimi passes through the most medial compartment.

51. Interossei of hand

(a) Palmar interossei abduct, while dorsal interossei adduct the digits.

(b) There are two dorsal interossei for the central finger.

(c) Usually all the interossei are supplied by deep branch of ulnar nerve.

(d) Dorsal interossei are bipinnate in nature.

(e) Paralysis of interossei leads to "claw hand" deformity.

52. Elbow joint

(a) It is a hinge (uniaxial) type of synovial joint.

(b) Anterior and posterior parts of capsule are very thin and weak.

(c) Medial collateral ligament is crossed by ulnar nerve.

(d) There is no communication between cavities of elbow and superior radioulnar joints.

(e) The base of lateral collateral ligament blends with annular ligament of superior radioulnar joint.

53. Radioulnar joint

(a) It is a pivot (uniaxial) type of synovial joint.

(b) Axis of pronation and supination passes through radial head, above and ulnar styloid process, below.

(c) Fibres of interosseous membrane descend obliquely towards postaxial bone (ulna).

(d) Forceful separation of radial head from capitulum of humerus, in adult individuals, is prevented mainly by quadrate ligament.

(e) Sometimes, inferior radioulnar joint communicates with wrist joint through a perforation in the triangular articular disc.

54. Wrist joint

(a) It is an ellipsoid (biaxial) type of synovial joint.

(b) Because of lower level of ulnar styloid process, the range of adduction is greater than that of abduction.

(c) It is essentially a radiocarpal joint as ulna does not participate in the articulation.

(d) At the end of adduction, triquetral comes to lie in contact with the triangular articular disc.

(e) Intra-articular injections in the joint are preferably given from the medial side.

LOWER LIMB

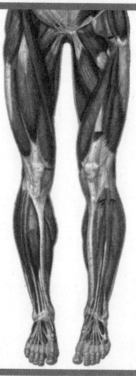

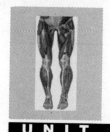

LOWER LIMB

Find out incorrect statement in each set.

55. Development of lower limb

(a) Limb buds appear at the end of 4th week of intrauterine life.

(b) Hindlimb appears few days later than the forelimb.

(c) The mesenchymal core of the limb is derived from splanchnopleuric mesoderm.

(d) Interdigital clefts appear as a result of death of mesenchymal cells, their removal by phagocytosis and invagination of surface ectoderm.

(e) After rotation, medial and lateral borders of lower limb represent its pre- and postaxial borders, respectively.

56. Hip bone

(a) Its three constituents, ilium, ischium and pubis, meet at acetabulum to form a V-shaped junction.

(b) Primary centres for ilium, ischium and pubis appear in 2nd, 3rd and 4th months of intrauterine life, respectively.

(c) Posterior superior iliac spine lies 4 cm lateral to 2nd sacral spine.

(d) Compact bone is maximum along arcuate line, which represents the line of weight transmission from sacrum to head of femur.

(e) Body weight is transmitted through lower medial part of ischial tuberosity, in sitting posture.

57. Femur

(a) Its head is directed upwards, medially and slightly forwards.

(b) Its lateral condyle projects more forwards than its medial condyle, providing stability to the patella.

(c) Calcar femorale, a thin plate of bone, extends from region of linea aspcera to the neck and greater trochanter of femur.

(d) Vastus intermedius is attached to front and medial surface of the femoral shaft.

(e) Appearance of the secondary centre at its lower end is a reliable indication of a full term baby, and hence of great medicolegal importance.

58. Tibia

(a) Its medial surface is subcutaneous and hence it is easily approachable surgically.

(b) Lack of muscular attachment in the lower part of tibia is responsible for its relative avascularity and hence difficult healing in case of the fracture.

(c) Epiphyseal lines at its both the ends are outside the adjacent joint cavities and thus the infections in the metaphyses rarely involve the corresponding joints.

(d) Its anterior border provides attachment to interosseous membrane.

(e) Its lateral surface provides attachment to the tibialis anterior.

59. Fibula

(a) Muscles of all the three compartments of leg get attached to the fibula.

(b) The appearance of the secondary centre and its fusion with the shaft take place earlier at its upper end than at its lower end.

(c) Malleolar fossa faces backwards and medially.

(d) Nutrient canal is directed downwards.

(e) Common peroneal nerve winds round the lateral aspect of the fibular neck.

60. Skeleton of foot

(a) Tarsal bones each have one centre of ossification, except calcaneus which has an additional scale-like epiphysis posteriorly.

(b) Out of five metatarsals, the 2nd one is the commonest to fracture as its base is relatively fixed.

(c) Sustentaculum tali is a projection from talus.

(d) Distal surface of calcaneus articulates with cuboid.

(e) Intermediate cuneiform is the smallest of three cuneiforms.

61. Cutaneous innervation of thigh

(a) The compression of lateral cutaneous nerve of thigh may be responsible for meralgia paraesthetica (pain on the lateral side of thigh).

(b) Posterior cutaneous nerve of thigh itself remains deep to deep fascia in the thigh, but its branches become cutaneous to supply along the posterior midline.

(c) Medial side of thigh is partly supplied by subsartorial plexus.

(d) Skin over the patella is supplied by 3rd lumbar spinal segment.

(e) Most of the cutaneous nerves for the front of thigh are derived from anterior division of obturator nerve.

62. Lymphatic drainage of the lower limb

(a) Most of the superficial lymphatics drain into lateral group of horizontal chain of superficial inguinal lymph nodes.

(b) Superficial lymphatics accompany the veins, while the deep lymphatics run along with the arteries.

(c) Deep lymphatics from foot and leg drain into the popliteal lymph nodes.

(d) Superficial lymphatics from lateral margin of foot and heel empty into the popliteal lymph nodes.

(e) One of the deep inguinal lymph nodes lying in the femoral canal, called lymph node of Cloquet, drains glans penis/clitoris.

63. Venous drainage of the lower limb

(a) Great saphenous vein is the longest vein in the body.

(b) Great saphenous vein, in front of medial malleolus, is commonly selected for "cut down" operation.

(c) The contraction of soleus plays an important role in venous return, hence it is also called the peripheral heart.

(d) Small saphenous vein is accompanied by posterior cutaneous nerve of thigh, in the upper half of leg.

(e) Incompetent valves in communicating veins result into flow of blood from superficial to deep.

64. Fascia lata

(a) Iliotibial tract is a thickened band on its anterior aspect.

(b) Cribriform fascia, a thin and weak site in it, is perforated by great saphenous vein, lymphatics and some superficial arteries.

(c) All the three intermuscular septa, medial, posterior and lateral, extend from its deep surface to the linea aspera of femur.

(d) It splits to enclose two muscles—tensor fasciae latae and gluteus maximus.

(e) It prevents bulging of muscles and maintains contour of the thigh.

65. Femoral triangle

(a) Inguinal ligament forms its base, whereas medial margins of sartorius and adductor longus form its lateral and medial borders, respectively.

(b) Iliopsoas, pectineus and adductor longus lie in its floor.

(c) Femoral canal, a potential space in the medial part of the femoral sheath, is the site for femoral hernia.

(d) Between pectineus and adductor longus, adductor brevis and anterior division of obturator nerve can be observed.

(e) The lateral part of femoral sheath is occupied by femoral vein, while in its intermediate part lie femoral artery and femoral branch of genitofemoral nerve.

66. Femoral artery

(a) It is the continuation of external iliac artery beyond the inguinal ligament and continues as popliteal artery beyond the hiatus magnus.

(b) Its superficial and deep external pudendal branches run medially superficial and deep to the spermatic cord (in males) or round ligament of uterus (in females), respectively.

(c) Rarely it splits and reunites before passing through the hiatus magnus.

(d) It can be most effectively compressed against the body of the pubis.

(e) It is represented by upper two-thirds of a line joining the midinguinal point and adductor tubercle.

67. The femoral nerve

(a) It is the largest branch of lumbar plexus.

(b) It is derived from the ventral divisions of the ventral rami of 2nd, 3rd and 4th lumbar nerves.

(c) It enters the thigh behind the inguinal ligament and lies lateral to the femoral sheath.

(d) It gives of muscular (extensor compartment of thigh), cutaneous (front of thigh and medial aspects of leg and foot), vascular (femoral artery and its branches) and articular (knee and hip joints) branches.

(e) Between its two divisions runs the lateral circumflex femoral artery.

68. Muscles of extensor compartment of thigh

(a) Out of the four components, i.e. vastus medialis, vastus intermedius, vastus lateralis and rectus femoris, the former three arise from the femur while the fourth one arises by its two (straight and oblique) heads from the ilium.

(b) Patella is the sesamoid bone developing in the tendon of quadriceps femoris.

(c) Quadriceps femoris is specially active during walking uphill.

(d) The lower fibres of vastus medialis, attached to medial margin of patella, stabilize the latter during extension at knee.

(e) Sartorius causes flexion of leg and flexion, abduction and medial rotation of thigh.

69. Muscles of adductor compartment of thigh

(a) Rider's bone is the sesamoid bone developing in the tendon of adductor longus near its attachment to the body of the pubis.

(b) Adductor magnus is the most extensive of all the three adductors and receives its innervation from two sources (posterior division of obturator and tibial component of sciatic nerves).

(c) In addition to adduction, the three adductors also cause lateral rotation of thigh.

(d) Gracilis extends from ischiopubic rami to upper part of medial aspect of tibia and acts as a guy-rope along with sartorius and semitendinosus to support the pelvis.

(e) Adductor longus is sandwiched between femoral and profunda femoris arteries, while adductor brevis lies between the two (anterior and posterior) divisions of obturator nerve.

70. Adductor (Subsartorial or Hunter's) canal

(a) It is represented by middle third of a line joining midinguinal point and adductor tubercle.

(b) The adductor canal is roofed medially by an aponeurosis lying deep to the sartorius, while its anterior and posterior walls are formed by vastus medialis and adductors (longus and magnus), respectively.

(c) Femoral vessels, saphenous nerve and nerve to vastus intermedius constitute the contents of the canal.

(d) Femoral artery throughout the canal lies sandwiched between femoral vein and saphenous nerve.

(e) Femoral artery can be compressed laterally against the femoral shaft.

71. Profunda femoris artery

(a) It arises from the femoral artery 10 cm below the inguinal ligament.

(b) It descends between the adductor longus and brevis along with anterior division of obturator nerve.

(c) The two circumflex femoral and the four perforating arteries are its only named branches.

(d) Its perforating branches pass laterally behind the femur under tendinous arches of adductor magnus to end in the vastus lateralis.

(e) Ascending and descending branches of the perforating arteries form a vertical chain of anastomoses on the back of thigh.

72. Obturator nerve

(a) It is derived from the ventral divisions of ventral rami of lumbar 2, 3 and 4 spinal segments.

(b) It terminates into its anterior and posterior divisions only after entering the thigh.

(c) The articular branches from its anterior and posterior divisions supply hip and knee joints, respectively and constitute the anatomical basis of referred pain in one joint from the other.

(d) Accessory obturator nerve (L_3, L_4) present in about 30% of individuals, usually supplies pectineus and hip joint.

(e) A cutaneous branch to subsartorial plexus and a vascular branch to the femoral artery is generally given off by its anterior division.

73. Gluteal region–I

(a) The gluteal region extends vertically from iliac crest to gluteal fold and horizontally from natal cleft to the line extending between anterior superior iliac spine and greater trochanter.

(b) Its upper medial quadrant is the most suitable site for intramuscular injections in the gluteal region.

(c) Cutaneous nerves converge in this region from all the sides.

(d) The gluteal fold is formed due to attachment of skin to the deep fascia and excessive fat in the region.

(e) Its lymphatics drain into horizontal group of superficial inguinal lymph nodes.

74. Gluteal region–II

(a) Gluteus maximus is most active at the extremes of hip movements.

(b) Piriformis is the key muscle under cover of gluteus maximus.

(c) Superior gemellus is supplied by nerve to quadratus femoris, while inferior gemellus is innervated by nerve to obturator internus.

(d) Quadratus femoris is a lateral rotator of thigh.

(e) Trendelenburg's sign is positive (i.e. the pelvis of normal side sags when the patient stands on the diseased leg) in cases of paralysis of gluteus medius and minimus.

75. Gluteal region–III

(a) Nerve to obturator internus shares a common root value (L_5, S_1, S_2) with inferior gluteal nerve, while nerve to quadratus femoris has a root value (L_4, L_5, S_1) in common with superior gluteal nerve.

(b) Superior gluteal nerve also supplies tensor fasciae latae, in addition to the glutei-medius and minimus.

(c) Inferior gluteal nerve is solely meant for gluteus maximus.

(d) Nerve to quadratus femoris descends deep to obturator internus with two gemelli to reach the deep surface of the quadratus femoris.

(e) Nerve to obturator internus lies most medially while entering the lesser sciatic foramen along with pudendal nerve and internal pudendal vessels.

76. Gluteal region–IV

(a) Internal pudendal vessels lie between pudendal nerve and nerve to obturator internus before enter the lesser sciatic foramen.

(b) Superior gluteal artery participates in the anastomoses related to anterior superior iliac spine and greater trochanter.

(c) Superior and inferior gluteal arteries enter the gluteal region above and below the piriformis, respectively.

(d) Inferior gluteal artery provides a branch to the cruciate anastomosis.

(e) Companion artery of the sciatic nerve (axial artery) springs from the superior gluteal artery.

77. Hamstring muscles

(a) All these muscles arise from the ischial tuberosity.

(b) Their innervation is derived from tibial component of the sciatic nerve.

(c) They descend and diverge to form upper boundaries of the popliteal fossa.

(d) They cause extension at hip (middle of the range) and flexion at knee.

(e) The short head of biceps femoris is included in the hamstring group of muscles.

78. Sciatic nerve

(a) Its root value is L_5, S_1–S_4.

(b) It is the thickest nerve in the body.

(c) An intramuscular injection in the gluteal region by an unskilled person may injure this nerve.

(d) It supplies all the muscles of leg and foot.

(e) When it divides at a higher lever in the pelvis, the common peroneal nerve generally pierces the piriformis near its lower margin to enter the gluteal region.

79. Arterial anastomoses

(a) Trochanteric and cruciate anastomoses are formed by branches of gluteal arteries, circumflex femoral arteries and the first perforating branch of profunda femoris artery.

(b) Branches from femoral, popliteal, anterior tibial and posterior tibial arteries form rich anastomoses around the knee.

(c) Anterior tibial artery contributes equally to medial and lateral malleolar arterial networks.

(d) Branches from lower end of the peroneal artery contribute to medial malleolar arterial network.

(e) Arterial anastomoses provide potential collateral channels during obstruction of the main arteries.

80. Popliteal fossa–I

(a) It is a diamond-shaped region at the back of the knee.

(b) Its roof is formed by the deep fascia (popliteal fascia) which is pierced by several cutaneous nerves and small saphenous vein.

(c) The femur, capsule of the knee joint and fascia covering the popliteus muscle contribute to its floor.

(d) Its upper lateral, and the two lower boundaries are formed by biceps femoris, and the two heads of gastrocnemius, respectively.

(e) Its upper medial boundary is formed by sartorius, adductor magnus and gracilis.

81. Popliteal fossa–II

(a) Popliteal vessels, tibial nerve and their branches constitute the most important contents of the fossa.

(b) Popliteal vein is the deepest of all its contents.

(c) Middle genicular vessels and nerve pierce the oblique popliteal ligament.

(d) Small saphenous vein pierces its roof to enter the popliteal vein.

(e) Almost all muscular branches for superficial muscles of flexor compartment of leg arise from tibial nerve before it leaves the popliteal fossa.

82. Cutaneous innervation of leg

(a) Posterior cutaneous nerve of thigh supplies the upper half of posterior midline of the leg.
(b) Sural nerve supplies the lower medial part of posterior aspect of the leg.
(c) Saphenous nerve, a branch of femoral nerve; innervates medial half of leg.
(d) Upper lateral half of leg is supplied by lateral cutaneous nerve of calf.
(e) Lower lateral part of front of leg is innervated by superficial peroneal nerve.

83. Retinacula of ankle

(a) Retinacula are thickened bands in deep fascia to hold tendons in their appropriate positions.
(b) There are two extensor (superior and inferior), two peroneal (superior and inferior) and one flexor retinacula in the region of ankle.
(c) All these retinacula get attached to calcaneus except superior extensor retinaculum.
(d) Proximal limb of the Y-shaped inferior extensor retinaculum blends medially with the plantar aponeurosis.
(e) Inferior peroneal retinaculum is continuous with the stem of inferior extensor retinaculum.

84. Extensor compartment of leg–I

(a) All these muscles arise from tibia except tibialis anterior, which originates from fibula.
(b) Tibialis anterior brings about dorsiflexion and inversion of foot.

    (c) Peroneus tertius is attached to 5th metatarsal and therefore acts as an effective evertor of foot.

    (d) Extensor hallucis longus and extensor digitorum longus are extensors of great toe and lateral four toes, respectively.

    (e) Extensor digitorum longus and peroneus tertius share a common synovial sheath.

85. Extensor compartment of leg–II

    (a) Deep peroneal nerve, a branch of common peroneal nerve, supplies all the muscles of extensor compartment.

    (b) Anterior tibial artery, a branch of popliteal artery, enters the extensor compartment through upper part of interosseous membrane.

    (c) Injury to deep peroneal nerve results into "foot drop".

    (d) Deep peroneal nerve lies medial to anterior tibial artery underneath superior extensor retinaculum.

    (e) Branches from anterior tibial artery participate in anastomoses both around knee and ankle.

86. Peroneal compartment of leg

    (a) All the three peronei—longus, brevis and tertius, constitute the peroneal compartment muscles.

    (b) All its muscles are supplied by superficial peroneal nerve.

    (c) Tendon of peroneus longus helps in maintaining the transverse arch of foot.

    (d) Peroneus brevis tendon grooves posterior aspect of lateral malleolus and is inserted on base of 5th metatarsal.

    (e) Arterial supply of peroneal compartment is derived from branches of peroneal artery, which itself remains in flexor compartment.

87. Flexor compartment of leg–I

    (a) The gastrocnemius, soleus and plantaris constitute this group of muscles.

(b) Tendons of all these muscles fuse to form tendocalcaneus, which is attached on middle of posterior surface of calcaneus.

(c) A small sesamoid bone, called "fabella", is frequently found in the lateral head of gastrocnemius.

(d) The strength of gastrocnemius is more while its range of movement is less than that of soleus.

(e) Soleus is also called "peripheral heart" due to its role in venous return.

88. Flexor compartment of leg–II

(a) The attachment of muscular fibres of the popliteus to the lateral meniscus is the factor preventing its rupture during flexion at knee.

(b) Tibialis posterior is attached to all the tarsal bones except the talus.

(c) Flexor hallucis longus plays an important role in propulsion.

(d) The pull of flexor digitorum longus is brought in line with toes by flexor accessorius (quadratus plantae).

(e) Back of medial malleolus is grooved by tendon of flexor hallucis longus.

89. Flexor compartment of leg–III

(a) Tibial nerve supplies all the muscles of flexor compartment of leg.

(b) Posterior tibial artery, one of terminal branches of popliteal artery, is the main artery of this compartment.

(c) Posterior tibial artery runs lateral to the tibial nerve under the flexor retinaculum to enter the sole.

(d) Medial calcanean artery and nerve arise from posterior tibial artery and tibial nerve, respectively just proximal to their divisions.

(e) Peroneal artery, a branch of posterior tibial artery remains in flexor compartment.

90. Dorsum of foot

(a) Dorsalis pedis artery is the continuation of anterior tibial artery beyond the ankle.

(b) In addition to supplying extensor digitorum brevis, deep peroneal nerve also innervates skin of 2nd interdigital cleft and adjacent sides of 2nd and 3rd toes.

(c) Extensor digitorum brevis extends from calcaneus to medial four toes.

(d) 2nd, 3rd and 4th dorsal metatarsal arteries arise directly from arcuate artery.

(e) Dorsalis pedis artery is important clinically as it can be palpated easily.

91. Fasciocutaneous layer of the sole

(a) Major portion of the sole is supplied by cutaneous branches arising from medial and lateral plantar nerves.

(b) Skin of the sole is very thick due to thickened dermis.

(c) The central deep fascia of the sole is very much thickened and known as plantar aponeurosis.

(d) Skin of the heel receives its innervation from medial calcanean nerves.

(e) The medial and lateral marginal skin of the sole is supplied by saphenous and sural nerves, respectively.

92. First muscular layer of the sole

(a) Out of the three muscles, abductor hallucis, flexor digitorum brevis and abductor digiti minimi, the last one has got most extensive attachment at origin.

(b) The tendons of flexor digitorum brevis go to lateral four toes.

(c) Flexor digitorum brevis and abductor hallucis are supplied by lateral plantar nerve.

(d) Flexor digitorum brevis is considered to be a detached part of soleus.

(e) Abductor digiti minimi is innervated by lateral plantar nerve.

93. Second muscular layer of the sole

(a) It includes long flexor tendons and muscles (flexor accessorius and lumbricals) attached to them.

(b) Flexor accessorius has two heads, medial-muscular, and lateral tendinous.

(c) Flexor accessorius is a special flexor of lateral four toes at full plantar flexion, when flexor digitorum longus becomes out of action.

(d) The medial two lumbricals are supplied by medial plantar nerve, while the lateral two are innervated by lateral plantar nerve.

(e) Flexor accessorius commonly receives its innervation from lateral plantar nerve.

94. Third muscular layer of the sole

(a) Like 1st muscular layer, this layer also consists of three muscles, namely, flexor hallucis brevis, adductor hallucis and flexor digiti minimi brevis.

(b) Flexor hallucis brevis receives its innervation from medial plantar nerve, whereas the remaining two muscles are supplied by lateral plantar nerve.

(c) Transverse head of adductor hallucis has no bony attachment.

(d) All these muscles are confined to distal half of foot.

(e) Flexor hallucis brevis has got dual origin.

95. Fourth muscular layer of the sole

(a) This layer comprises three plantar and four dorsal interossei.

(b) The axis of adduction and abduction of toes passes through the 2nd toe.

(c) Plantar interossei are adductors (PAD), while dorsal interossei are abductors (DAB).

(d) 1st and 2nd dorsal interossei act on great toe and 2nd toe, respectively.

(e) 1st, 2nd and 3rd plantar interossei act on lateral three toes.

96. Medial plantar nerve

(a) It passes first under abductor hallucis and then appears between it and flexor digitorum brevis.

(b) It supplies three muscles in total, one each in 1st, 2nd and 3rd muscular layers.

(c) It innervates medial two-thirds of the skin of the sole except heel.

(d) It innervates skin of the plantar aspect of medial 3 and 1/2 toes.

(e) Its cutaneous branches for the sole appear along the medial margin of plantar aponeurosis.

97. Lateral plantar nerve

(a) Its proximal part runs obliquely lateralwards between 2nd and 3rd muscular layers of the sole.

(b) Its distal part course medially in the concavity of plantar arch between 3rd and 4th layers of muscles of the sole.

(c) Its cutaneous branches supply plantar aspects of lateral one and half toes.

(d) Its cutaneous branches for lateral one-third of the sole appear along the lateral margin of plantar aponeurosis.

(e) All the muscles of the sole, except flexor digitorum brevis, abductor hallucis, flexor hallucis brevis and 1st lumbrical, are supplied by lateral plantar nerve.

98. Plantar arteries

(a) Plantar arteries lie outer to the corresponding plantar nerves.

(b) Plantar arch is formed by distal curved part of medial plantar artery.

(c) All the plantar metatarsal arteries appear from the plantar arch.

(d) Distal perforating arteries connect the plantar metatarsal arteries with their dorsal counterparts.

(e) The proper plantar digital artery to lateral side of the little toe arises from the beginning of the plantar arch.

99. Hip joint

(a) It is a ball and socket type of synovial joint.
(b) It is stabilized mainly by its strong ligaments.
(c) The long femoral neck is the factor responsible for increasing its range of movement.
(d) The capacity of its cavity is maximum when the thigh is flexed, abducted and medially rotated, the posture preferably adopted by patients suffering from painful inflammatory conditions of this joint.
(e) Pain may be referred from hip joint to knee joint, and vice versa as both the joints have a common source of innervation, i.e. L_2–L_4 (femoral and obturator nerves).

100. Knee joint

(a) It is a condylar type of synovial joint.
(b) Cruciate ligaments provide anteroposterior stability to this joint.
(c) Popliteus unlocks the extended knee to allow the initiation of its flexion.
(d) Fibular collateral ligament is quite free from the capsule of this joint.
(e) Lateral meniscus is commonly crushed between femur and tibia.

101. Tibiofibular articulations

(a) Superior tibiofibular joint is a fibrous joint.
(b) Fibres of interosseous membrane descend obliquely towards the postaxial bone (fibula).
(c) Interosseous membrane is pierced by anterior tibial artery in its upper part, and by the perforating branch of peroneal artery in its lower part.

(d) Inferior tibiofibular joint is an example of syndesmosis, a type of fibrous joint.

(e) There are three tibiofibular ligaments, anterior, posterior and interosseous, connecting lower ends of tibia and fibula.

102. Ankle joint

(a) It is a hinge type of synovial joint.

(b) Its lateral ligament consists of three components, anterior and posterior talofibular, and calcaneofibular ligaments.

(c) Anterior tibiotalar ligament is the deep part of medial (deltoid) ligament.

(d) Forceful eversion of foot may result into avulsion of medial malleolus without leading to rupture of the strong deltoid ligament.

(e) Plantar flexion is accompanied by eversion, while dorsiflexion by inversion.

103. Small joints of the foot

(a) Talocalcaneonavicular and subtalar joints are mainly involved in inversion and eversion of the foot.

(b) Axis of inversion and eversion passes through centres of calcaneus and head of talus.

(c) Both the tibialis—anterior and posterior are invertors, while all the three peronei—longus, brevis, and tertius are evertors.

(d) Metatarsophalangeal joints belong to ellipsoid type of synovial joints.

(e) Interphalangeal joints are condylar type of synovial joints.

104. Arches of the foot

(a) The transverse arch of foot is formed by cuboid, three cuneiforms and bases of metatarsal bones.

(b) Plantar calcaneonavicular (spring), long plantar and short plantar (plantar calcaneocuboid) ligaments and plantar aponeurosis are essential for maintaining the longitudinal arches of foot, in standing posture.

(c) Long flexor tendons and muscles of 1st layer of the sole play an important role in maintaining the longitudinal arches of the foot.

(d) When the arches of the foot are collapsed, the condition is called "club foot".

(e) Adaptation to uneven ground, propulsion, resilience of the foot and protection of nerves and vessels of the sole, are some of the important functions of arches of the foot.

THORAX

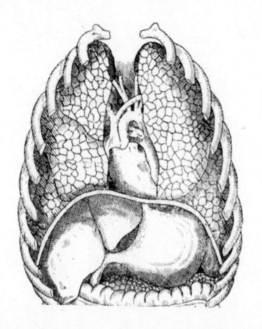

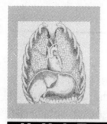

THORAX

Find out incorrect statement in each set.

105. Thorax framework

(a) It is a bellows-like chamber that moves during respiration.

(b) Its superior aperture is wider than its inferior one.

(c) Costal margin is contributed by the last two ribs and costal cartilages of 7th to 10th ribs.

(d) Of all the ribs, 7th is maximum in length while 9th is maximum in obliquity.

(e) The shape of the thorax is circular in cross-section in new-borns.

106. Sternum

(a) Its sides articulate with the upper seven costal cartilages to form the sternocostal joints, all of which are synovial in nature.

(b) It consists of three parts; manubrium, body and xiphoid process.

(c) Sternal foramen is occasionally present at the junction of 3rd and 4th sternebrae of its body.

(d) Sternal puncture is usually done for bone marrow examinations.

(e) The process of ossification in sternebrae progresses from above downwards, while its completion proceeds in reverse direction.

107. 1st rib

(a) It is the least curved rib.

(b) It is marked by scalene tubercle for the attachment of scalenus anterior, which is sandwiched between subclavian vessels.

(c) The front of its neck is crossed from medial to lateral by sympathetic chain, lst posterior intercostal vein, superior intercostal artery and T_1 root of brachial plexus.

(d) Its angle coincides with its tubercle.

(e) Its inner margin gives attachment to suprapleural membrane (Sibson's fascia).

108. 12th rib

(a) It is distinguished by its negative features, i.e. absence of neck, tubercle, angle and costal groove.

(b) The lateral part of its inner surface is related to the costal pleura.

(c) Its inner surface gives attachment to the lateral arcuate ligament.

(d) Its inner surface faces upwards as the chest is barrel-shaped.

(e) It provides attachment to the anterior and middle layers of thoracolumbar fascia and quadratus lumborum.

109. Typical rib

(a) It has a posterior end (consisting of head, neck and tubercle), a shaft and an anterior end.

(b) The lower facet of its head is larger than the upper one.

(c) The sharp upper border (crest) of its neck provides attachment to superior costotransverse ligament.

(d) The floor of its costal groove gives attachment to intercostalis intimus.

(e) Its angle (posterior) provides attachment to the upward continuation of thoracolumbar fascia.

110. Thoracic vertebrae

(a) The first and the last four thoracic vertebrae are atypical in nature.

(b) Vertebral column in the upper thoracic region often shows a lateral curvature.

(c) Of all the thoracic vertebrae, the 5th one has got the smallest body.

(d) The spines of the midthoracic vertebrae are directed almost vertically downwards, in comparison to their counterparts in the upper and lower thoracic regions.

(e) Their vertebral foramina are smaller than those of cervical and lumbar vertebrae.

111. Superior aperture of thorax

(a) It is kidney-shaped and measures about 5 cm anteroposteriorly and 10 cm transversely.

(b) Its boundaries are formed by the body of the 1st thoracic vertebra posteriorly, superior border of the manubrium sterni anteriorly and inner margins of the 1st pair of ribs on the sides.

(c) Its plane is horizontal.

(d) Its so called diaphragm (Sibson's fascia) is attached to inner border of the 1st rib and to anterior margin of transverse process of the 7th cervical vertebra.

(e) It is occupied in midline by oesophagus, trachea, thoracic duct and left recurrent laryngeal nerve and on each side by apex of the lung and cervical pleura.

112. Respiratory movements

(a) Pump handle movement increases the transverse diameter of the thorax.

(b) Contraction of the diaphragm increases the vertical diameter of the thorax.

(c) The flat articular surfaces of the lower costotransverse joints facilitate the bucket handle movement.

(d) In the newborns, the respiration is mainly of abdominal type.

(e) During inspiration, the costal cartilages become less oblique.

113. Inferior aperture of thorax

(a) It slopes obliquely downwards and backwards.

(b) Its boundaries are contributed by 12th thoracic vertebra, 12th ribs, costal cartilages of 7th to 12th ribs and sternum.

(c) It is closed by a fibromuscular partition, called the diaphragm.

(d) During deep inspiration, its level is raised up.

(e) It is narrower transversely than anteroposteriorly.

114. Intercostal muscle

(a) External intercostal muscle extends from tubercle of rib to the costochondral junction.

(b) The interchondral fibres of internal intercostal muscle together with external intercostal muscle assist inspiration, while intercostal fibres of the former facilitate expiration.

(c) In case of paralysis of intercostal muscles, there occurs bulging in the corresponding space during expiration.

(d) The 3rd (deepest) layer of intercostal muscles consists of intercostalis intimus only.

(e) The internal intercostal muscle runs from the floor of costal groove of the rib above to the upper border of the rib below.

115. Intercostal nerves

(a) The ventral rami of all the thoracic spinal nerves, except the 12th one, continue as intercostal nerves.

(b) The 1st intercostal nerve usually supplies no skin as it lacks both lateral, and anterior terminal cutaneous branches.

(c) The lateral cutaneous branch of 2nd intercostal nerve (intercostobrachial nerve) supplies the floor of axilla and upper medial part of the arm.

(d) To avoid injury to the intercostal nerve, a clinician should introduce the needle near the lower border of the rib.

(e) The collateral branch of an intercostal nerve, if present, courses along the lower border of intercostal space to supply the intercostal muscles.

116. Intercostal arteries

(a) All the posterior intercostal arteries arise from descending thoracic aorta except the 1st two, which are derived from superior intercostal artery.

(b) The dilatation of intercostal artery is responsible for the erosion of the corresponding rib in cases of coarctation of aorta.

(c) For each of upper 6 intercostal spaces, the internal thoracic artery while for each of the next 3 spaces, the musculophrenic artery, give off two anterior intercostal arteries.

(d) Internal thoracic artery is ligated preferably in the 4th intercostal space.

(e) Intercostal artery remains sandwiched between the corresponding vein and nerve, during its course.

117. Intercostal veins

(a) The anterior intercostal veins accompany the corresponding arteries to drain into internal thoracic vein(s) or musculophrenic veins.

(b) First (highest) posterior intercostal vein on each side crosses the neck of the 1st rib to join the corresponding brachiocephalic vein.

(c) On the left side, posterior intercostal veins of 4th to 8th intercostal spaces join the accessory hemiazygos vein, while those of 9th to 11th spaces join the hemiazygos vein.

(d) On the right side, all the posterior intercostal veins, except the 1st one, drain into the azygos vein.

(e) Both, hemiazygos and accessory hemiazygos veins cross the body of 6th thoracic vertebra to enter the azygos vein.

118. Mediastinum

(a) It is a movable median septum between the two pleural cavities.

(b) The superior mediastinum is separated from the inferior one by a plane passing between 2nd and 3rd thoracic vertebrae.

(c) The fibrous pericardium divides the inferior mediastinum into three parts—anterior, middle and posterior.

(d) DOVA, i.e. duct (thoracic), oesophagus, veins (azygos and hemiazygos) and aorta (descending thoracic) constitute the main contents of the posterior mediastinum.

(e) Posterior mediastinum communicates with the abdomen through the aortic hiatus.

119. Pleura

(a) The pleural cavity is a potential space between the parietal and visceral layers of pleura.

(b) A narrow fascial band, called phrenicopleural fascia, keeps the pleura of costodiaphragmatic recess in place during respiration.

(c) Visceral pleura is sensitive to pain.

(d) In the pleural cavity, there may occur accumulation of air (pneumothorax), clear fluid (hydrothorax), pus (pyothorax) or blood (haemothorax).

(e) The peripheral diaphragmatic and costal pleurae are supplied by the intercostal nerves, while the central diaphragmatic and mediastinal pleurae are innervated by the phrenic nerve.

120. Root of the lung

(a) It consists of the structures which enter or leave the hilum of the lung.

(b) Its most anterior structure is the superior pulmonary vein.

(c) Its lowest structure, the inferior pulmonary vein, is free to dilate and move in the pulmonary ligament.

(d) The right primary bronchus divides into eparterial and hyparterial bronchi, which enter the lung above and below the pulmonary artery, respectively.

(e) It is arched by azygos vein on the left side and arch of aorta on the right side.

121. Thoracic part of sympathetic trunk

(a) It consists of only 11 ganglia in more than 70% of individuals.

(b) Preganglionic section of its upper part is preferred to treat the Raynaud's disease involving upper limb.

(c) Greater, lesser and least splanchnic nerves emerge from 5th to 8th, 9th to 10th, and 11th thoracic ganglia, respectively.

(d) Its ganglia are connected to the ventral rami of the corresponding spinal nerves by grey rami communicans only.

(e) First thoracic ganglion frequently fuses with the inferior cervical ganglion to form the stellate (cervicothoracic) ganglion.

122. Vena azygos

(a) It commences in the abdomen and enters the thorax through the aortic hiatus.

(b) It drains into the superior vena cava.

(c) It commonly receives the right superior intercostal vein.

(d) It is provided with a number of competent valves.

(e) It is crossed posteriorly by the right posterior intercostal arteries arising from the descending thoracic aorta.

123. Phrenic nerve

(a) Its root value is cervical 3, 4 and 5 spinal segments.

(b) It descends usually behind the subclavian artery.

(c) It is a mixed nerve.

(d) It accompanies pericardiacophrenic branch of internal thoracic artery in the thorax.

(e) Phrenicotomy is done occasionally to reduce the expansion of the diseased lung, in cases of pulmonary tuberculosis.

124. Lungs

(a) The right lung is broader, shorter and heavier than the left one.

(b) The left lung is commonly characterized by the cardiac notch.

(c) Anomalous azygos lobe may be present in the left lung.

(d) The right lung is usually divided into 3 lobes, while the left one into 2 lobes only.

(e) The apex of the lung may be involved in cases of perforating wounds above the level of thoracic inlet.

125. Bronchi

(a) The right and left bronchi are 2.5 cm and 5.0 cm in length, respectively.

(b) The tertiary bronchi are ten in number on the right side, while only eight or nine on the left side.

(c) Foreign body commonly enters the right principal bronchus due to its wider lumen and more vertical position.

(d) A "subapical" segment is present in the upper lobe of the right lung in more than 50% of the individuals.

(e) The right principal bronchus passes below the arch of vena azygos while the left one runs below the arch of aorta.

126. Blood vessels of lung

(a) The pulmonary arteries and their branches closely follow the bronchial tree.

(b) The pulmonary veins (superior and inferior) carry oxygenated blood to the left atrium.

(c) The pulmonary arteries carry deoxygenated blood to the alveoli, while the bronchial arteries supply oxygenated blood to the rest of the lung.

(d) Two left bronchial arteries (upper and lower) arise from the front of the descending thoracic aorta, while only one right bronchial artery commonly originates from 3rd right posterior intercostal artery.

(e) The main bronchial vessels run on the ventral aspect of the extrapulmonary bronchi.

127. Lymph nodes and lymphatics of lung

(a) Superficial and deep lymphatics converge towards the bronchopulmonary (hilar) lymph nodes, which lie in the hilum of the lung.

(b) Pulmonary lymph nodes are found in the substance of the lung close to its hilum.

(c) Efferents of tracheobronchial lymph nodes enter the bronchopulmonary group of lymph nodes.

(d) The bronchomediastinal trunk usually opens into the corresponding brachiocephalic vein.

(e) The bronchogenic carcinoma (responsible for about one-third of all cancer deaths in men) spreads rapidly to the tracheobronchial and mediastinal lymph nodes and may involve the recurrent laryngeal nerve.

128. Anterior mediastinum

(a) It is bounded anteriorly by the body of the sternum and posteriorly by the pericardium.

(b) It contains part of thymus, a few lymph nodes, some mediastinal branches of internal thoracic artery, two sternopericardial ligaments and loose areolar tissue.

(c) Thymus is derived from the 2nd pharyngeal pouch (endodermal).

(d) Thymus is nearly as large as the heart in the newborns, but is greatly reduced in size after puberty.

(e) Thymus derives its blood supply originally from the inferior thyroid artery, which is replaced later on during the descent by the internal thoracic artery.

129. Pericardium

(a) The fibrous pericardium is derived from the septum transversum.

(b) The base of the fibrous pericardium corresponds with the base of the heart.

(c) The oblique sinus is a blind recess behind the left atrium between right and left pulmonary veins.

(d) The fibrous pericardium and parietal layer of the serous pericardium are supplied by the phrenic nerve, whereas the visceral layer of the serous pericardium receives autonomic innervation.

(e) The arterial supply of the visceral layer of the serous pericardium is derived from the coronary arteries.

130. Sternocostal surface of the heart

(a) Superficial cardiac dullness marks the sternocostal surface of the heart, which is not covered by the lungs.

(b) The right border of the heart lies about 4 cm lateral to the right sternal margin.

(c) The apex beat is usually palpated in the left 5th intercostal space just medial to the midclavicular (mammary) line.

(d) Pulmonary and aortic valves lie at the level of 3rd costal cartilage and 3rd intercostal space, respectively.

(e) Bicuspid (mitral) valve is located behind the left half of sternum at the level of 4th costal cartilage, while tricuspid valve is situated at the level of 4th intercostal space behind the right half of sternum.

131. Coronary arteries

(a) The right coronary artery is commonly larger in diameter than the left one.

(b) The sinuatrial and atrioventricular nodes are commonly supplied by nodal branches of the right coronary artery.

(c) The right and left coronary arteries arise from the anterior and left posterior aortic sinuses, respectively.

(d) The descending branch of the left coronary artery is the commonest to be involved in the myocardial infarction.

(e) The coronary arteries and their major branches usually run deep to the visceral layer of the serous pericardium.

132. Veins of the heart

(a) The coronary sinus, about 3 cm in length, lies in the posterior part of the coronary sulcus.

(b) The anterior cardiac veins drain directly into the right atrium.

(c) The venae cordis minimae (Thebesian veins) open directly into the chambers of the heart particularly into right atrium and right ventricle.

(d) Thé oblique vein of left atrium (of Marshall) is the remnant of distal part of left vitelline vein.

(e) The blood flow in the proximal part of great cardiac vein, and in the circumflex artery is in the same direction.

133. Nerves of the heart

(a) A cardiac ganglion is usually present in the superficial cardiac plexus, situated below the arch of aorta and to the right of ligamentum arteriosum.

(b) Its sympathetic fibres are acceleratory, while parasympathetic fibres are inhibitory to the heart.

(c) All the cardiac branches derived from sympathetic chains, vagi and recurrent laryngeal nerves contribute to the deep cardiac plexus-except:

(i) left superior cervical sympathetic, cardiac nerve and

(ii) left inferior cervical vagal cardiac nerve.

(d) Afferents for cardiac pain travel in all sympathetic cardiac nerves.

(e) The right coronary plexus is formed by both superficial and deep cardiac plexuses, while the left coronary plexus is derived chiefly from the prolongation of left half of deep cardiac plexus.

134. Right atrium

(a) Sulcus terminalis on its surface corresponds with the crista terminalis, a vertical muscular ridge at the junction of anterior rough and posterior smooth parts of its chamber.

(b) Limbus fossa ovalis is the crescentic upper margin of fossa ovalis in its posterior wall.

(c) Atrioventricular node lies deep to its triangle of Koch, which is bounded by septal leaf of tricuspid valve, coronary sinus orifice and tendon of Todaro.

(d) The coronary sinus opens into it between right atrioventricular orifice and opening of superior vena cava.

(e) Openings in the right atrium are right atrioventricular orifice, openings of superior and inferior venae cavae, coronary sinus, anterior cardiac veins and venae cordis minimae.

135. Superior vena cava

(a) It receives blood from upper half of the body.

(b) It is formed by the union of two brachiocephalic veins opposite the upper border of right 1st costal cartilage and enters the right atrium at the level of lower border of right 3rd costal cartilage.

(c) Its lower half is contained within the fibrous pericardium.

(d) It is derived from right common cardinal and right anterior cardinal veins.

(e) Azygos vein joins its posterior aspect at the level of sternal angle of Louis.

136. Right ventricle

(a) It receives blood from the right atrium, and pumps it into the pulmonary trunk.

(b) The thickness of its wall is 3 times of the left ventricular wall.

(c) Its rough part, having trabeculae carnae, is derived from the primitive ventricular chamber.

(d) Its upper part (the infundibulum) is marked by abundance of fibroelastic tissue.

(e) Moderator band (septomarginal trabecula) provides passage to the right branch of the atrioventricular bundle of His.

137. Pulmonary trunk

(a) It is approximately 5 cm in length, 3 cm in diameter, and is contained within the fibrous pericardium.

(b) It lies first in front and then to the right of the ascending aorta.

(c) It is the common site for embolism, which may result into respiratory distress and prove fatal.

(d) It terminates into right and left pulmonary arteries at the level of angle of Louis.

(e) The pulmonary valve has three cusps, two anterior (right and left) and one posterior.

138. Left ventricle

(a) It contributes to the sternocostal, left and diaphragmatic surfaces and the apex of the heart.

(b) The blood pressure in the left ventricle is 6 times higher than that in the right ventricle.

(c) Its aortic vestibule is mainly muscular and contractile in nature.

(d) Mitral valve has got an anterior larger and a posterior smaller cusp.

(e) In addition to separating the two ventricles from each other, membranous part of the interventricular septum also intervenes between right atrium and left ventricle.

139. Ascending aorta

(a) It is approximately 5.0 cm in length.

(b) It is an elastic artery.

(c) No branch arises from it.

(d) Aortic bulb is the bulging from the right side of the junction of ascending aorta and arch of aorta.

(e) It is situated mainly opposite the highest sternebra of the body of the sternum.

140. Brachiocephalic veins

(a) Each begins behind the medial end of the corresponding clavicle.

(b) The two brachiocephalic veins unite to form the superior vena cava at the lower border of right 1st costal cartilage.

(c) Internal thoracic, vertebral, inferior thyroid and 1st posterior (highest) intercostal veins are the only tributaries of each of them.

(d) The lengths of right and left brachiocephalic veins are about 3.5 and 6.5 cm, respectively.

(e) The left brachiocephalic vein runs downwards and to the right just above the arch of aorta, crossing its branches superficially.

141. Arch of aorta

(a) It arches over the root of the left lung behind the upper half of manubrium sterni.

(b) Its right posterior aspect is related to trachea, oesophagus and left recurrent laryngeal nerve.

(c) It is crossed by left phrenic and left vagus nerves on its left anterior aspect.

(d) It gives off 3 large branches (brachiocephalic, left common carotid and left subclavian arteries) from its upper convexity.

(e) Its narrowing (coarctation), if present, is commonly located in close relationship with ligamentum arteriosum, the fibrous remnant of ductus arteriosus.

142. Pulmonary arteries

(a) The right pulmonary artery is slightly larger than the left one.

(b) They enter the lungs behind the corresponding upper pulmonary veins.

(c) Inside the lungs, their branches follow the pattern of the bronchial tree.

(d) They carry oxygenated blood and supply nutrition to whole of the lungs.

(e) Ligamentum arteriosum and the ligament of left vena cava are attached to the left pulmonary artery.

143. Left atrium

(a) It is situated behind, to the left, and slightly above the right atrium.

(b) Its smooth part is derived from the primitive atrium, while its rough part develops by incorporation of the pulmonary veins.

(c) It receives oxygenated blood from the lungs through pulmonary veins.

(d) It communicates with the left ventricle through the left atrioventricular orifice.

(e) It is related posteriorly to oblique sinus, fibrous pericardium and oesophagus.

144. Myocardium and conducting system of the heart

(a) Muscle fibres in atria and ventricles run in two layers, superficial and deep.

(b) The only continuity between atrial and ventricular musculature is through the atrioventricular bundle of His.

(c) Sinuatrial node is subepicardial and is situated at the upper end of sulcus terminalis near the right margin of opening of superior vena cava.

(d) Atrioventricular node is located just above the opening of coronary sinus in the right atrium.

(e) Purkinje fibres are subepicardial in position.

145. Thoracic part of trachea

(a) It is confined to the superior mediastinum.

(b) C-shaped tracheal rings of hyaline cartilage occupy the posterior aspect and sides of the trachea leaving a gap anteriorly, filled by the muscle trachealis.

(c) The entire trachea is supplied by inferior thyroid arteries except the part near its bifurcation, which receives its supply from the bronchial arteries.

(d) During its descent, it deviates slightly from the midline to the right side.

(e) Its immediate posterior relation is formed by the oesophagus.

146. Cardiac plexus

(a) Its preganglionic sympathetic neurons are located in the intermediolateral column of middle 4 (5th to 8th) thoracic segments of the spinal cord.

(b) Superficial cardiac plexus is formed by the upper cervical cardiac branch of left sympathetic trunk and lower cervical cardiac branch of the left vagus.

(c) Deep cardiac plexus is situated in front of bifurcation of the trachea and behind the arch of aorta.

(d) Both the cardiac plexuses, superficial and deep, contribute to the right coronary plexus.

(e) Its sympathetic fibres are coronary dilator in nature.

147. Thoracic part of the vagus nerves

(a) The right vagus is closely applied to the trachea, while the left one is separated from it by arch of aorta.

(b) The cardiac, pulmonary and oesophageal branches arise from both the vagi to supply the corresponding viscera.

(c) The left recurrent laryngeal nerve arises from the left vagus in the thorax and hooks round inferior surface of the arch of aorta behind the attachment of ligamentum arteriosum.

(d) The vagi descend and break up in front of the corresponding roots of lungs to form pulmonary plexuses along with sympathetic twigs from 2nd, 3rd and 4th thoracic sympathetic ganglia.

(e) Anterior and posterior vagal trunks are derived mainly from left and right vagus nerves, respectively, though each gets contributions from both the vagi.

148. Pulmonary plexus

(a) The anterior and posterior pulmonary plexuses are situated in relation to the corresponding aspects of root of the lung.

(b) Its sympathetic and parasympathetic fibres are derived from 2nd to 5th thoracic sympathetic ganglia and vagus nerve, respectively.

(c) The left posterior pulmonary plexus receives additional fibres from the left recurrent laryngeal nerve.

(d) Its branches follow and supply the bronchial tree and accompanying arteries.

(e) Its sympathetic fibres are bronchoconstrictor and vasodilator in nature.

149. Oesophagus

(a) It measures about 25 cm in length.

(b) It extends from 6th cervical to 11th thoracic vertebral levels.

(c) It does not show any curvature.

(d) Its anterior wall is indented by arch of aorta, left bronchus and left atrium from above downwards.

(e) It enters the abdomen at the level of 10th thoracic vertebra through the oesophageal hiatus of the diaphragm.

150. Thoracic duct

(a) It drains lymph from the whole body except right halves of head, neck and thorax, and right upper limb.

(b) It begins at the upper end of cisterna chyli which lies in front of the 1st and 2nd lumbar vertebrae.

(c) It enters the thorax through the aortic hiatus between descending aorta and azygos vein.

(d) It opens into the commencement of the left brachiocephalic vein between the corresponding internal jugular and subclavian veins.

(c) It does not have any valve.

151. Lymphatic drainage of the thoracic viscera

(a) Tracheobronchial lymph nodes which drain the lungs form five main groups, namely, paratracheal, superior tracheo-bronchial, inferior tracheobronchial, bronchopulmonary and pulmonary lymph nodes.

(b) Lymphatics from the heart drain into inferior tracheobronchial and brachiocephalic lymph nodes.

(c) Most of the lymphatics from the oesophagus enter the posterior mediastinal lymph nodes.

(d) Lymphatics from the thymus end in the brachiocephalic, tracheobronchial and parasternal lymph nodes.

(e) In primary pulmonary tuberculosis, the tracheobronchial group of lymph nodes are rarely infected.

152. Sternal and sternocostal joints

(a) Manubriosternal joint is a secondary cartilaginous joint (symphysis).

(b) The 1st sternocostal articulation is a primary cartilaginous joint (synchondrosis).

(c) All the sternocostal joints from 2nd to 7th are of synovial type with a single joint cavity.

(d) In pump handle movement, the sternum moves upwards and forwards and makes the sternal angle more prominent.

(e) Xiphisternal joint usually ossifies by the age of 40 years.

153. Costovertebral joints

(a) Posterior end of a typical rib articulates by the synovial joints with transverse process and body of the corresponding vertebra as well as with the body of the vertebra above.

(b) The head of a typical rib has got a lower larger facet for the body of the corresponding vertebra and an upper smaller facet for the body of the vertebra above.

(c) Bucket handle movement is facilitated by upper costo-transverse joints.

(d) Posterior end of the rib is connected to the transverse process of the corresponding vertebra by costotransverse and lateral costotransverse ligaments, and to that of vertebra above by superior costotransverse ligament.

(e) The cavity of the most of the joints of the heads of ribs is divided into two compartments by an intra-articular ligament.

BRAIN

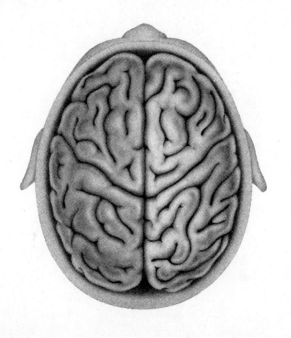

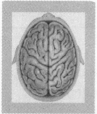

BRAIN

Find out incorrect statement in each set.

154. Brain development

(a) It is ectodermal in origin except its microglia which are derived from the mesoderm.

(b) The cephalic dilatation of the neural tube develops into brain whereas its caudal narrow portion becomes the spinal cord.

(c) Three primary cerebral vesicles; prosencephalon, mesencephalon and metencephalon grow to form forebrain, midbrain and hindbrain, respectively.

(d) Both cephalic (midbrain) and cervical flexures have a ventral concavity, while pontine flexure shows a ventral convexity.

(e) Neurons of the mantle zone migrate towards the surfaces of cerebrum and cerebellum to give rise to their cortices.

155. Neuron

(a) It is the structural and functional unit of the nervous system.

(b) Its soma (perikaryon) is marked by the presence of nucleus and Nissl substance.

(c) Its dendrites differ from its axons due to the lack of branching and Nissl substance.

(d) Its dendrites carry impulses towards its soma.

(e) In adult brain, the neurons are postmitotic cells.

156. Neuroglia

(a) Neuroglia are 10 times more numerous than the neurons.
(b) Fibrous astrocytes are present mainly in the grey matter.
(c) Microglia behave like macrophages.
(d) Oligodendrocytes are the source of myelin sheaths in the central nervous system.
(e) Neuroglia possess the mitotic potential even in the adult brain.

157. Parts of the brain

(a) The brain is divisible into forebrain, midbrain and hindbrain.
(b) Midbrain, pons and medulla together constitute the brainstem.
(c) Cerebellum, pons and medulla together constitute the hindbrain.
(d) The forebrain consists of the two cerebral hemispheres only.
(e) Diencephalon consists of thalamus, hypothalamus, subthalamus, epithalamus and metathalamus.

158. Dura mater

(a) It is the outermost and a tough covering of the brain.
(b) It consists of an inner meningeal and an outer endosteal layer.
(c) Falx cerebri, falx cerebelli, tentorium cerebelli and diaphragm sellae are formed by the duplication of its meningeal layer.
(d) It is ectodermal in origin.
(e) Its innervation is derived from trigeminal and upper three cervical nerves, and cervical sympathetic trunk.

159. Arachnoid mater

(a) It is derived largely from the neural crest.
(b) Its protrusions in dural venous sinuses form arachnoid villi and granulations.
(c) It is separated from the pia mater by subarachnoid space filled with cerebrospinal fluid.
(d) Delicate fibrous strands (trabeculae) connect it with the pia mater.

(e) Arachnoid mater and dura mater are usually pierced by the cranial nerves at different points.

160. Cerebrospinal fluid

(a) It provides buoyancy to the brain.
(b) It is derived from the choroid plexuses and the ependyma.
(c) Its volume is greatly reduced from the normal (130 to 150 ml), in cases of the hydrocephalus.
(d) It is drained by the arachnoid villi and granulations.
(e) It is obtained by lumbar or cisternal puncture for investigative purposes.

161. Pia mater

(a) It is largely derived from the neural crest.
(b) Its invagination into a brain ventricle is called tela choroidea.
(c) It loosely covers the brain surfaces and bridges over the sulci.
(d) It bounds the perivascular space around the arterial twigs entering the brain.
(e) It is highly vascular particularly in the regions of choroid plexuses.

162. Superficial veins of cerebrum

(a) Superior cerebral veins open into the superior sagittal sinus obliquely forward against the current of the blood in the sinus.
(b) Superior and inferior anastomotic veins connect the posterior end of the superficial middle cerebral vein with the superior sagittal and transverse sinuses, respectively.
(c) Superficial middle cerebral vein joins the basal vein.
(d) Inferior surface of cerebrum is drained by sphenoparietal, cavernous, superior petrosal, transverse and straight sinuses.
(e) Superior cerebral veins drain the greater parts of superolateral as well as medial surfaces of the cerebrum.

163. Deep veins of cerebrum

(a) Basal vein is formed by the union of anterior cerebral, striate and superficial middle cerebral veins.

(b) Basal veins wind round the midbrain to end in the great cerebral vein (of Galen).

(c) Internal cerebral vein is formed by the union of the thalamostriate and choroidal veins.

(d) Each internal cerebral vein begins at the interventricular foramen and ends into the great cerebral vein.

(e) Great cerebral vein passes below the splenium of corpus callosum and joins the inferior sagittal sinus to form the straight sinus.

164. Circle of Willis

(a) It lies in the interpeduncular fossa around the optic chiasma and the pituitary stalk.

(b) It is formed by two cerebral (anterior and posterior), two communicating (anterior and posterior) arteries along with the internal carotid arteries.

(c) In majority (60%) of the cases, circle of Willis shows anomalies.

(d) It equalizes the blood pressure on the two sides of the brain during different positions of the head.

(e) The collateral circulation in circle of Willis is always adequate enough to prevent the hemiplegia of the opposite side, if one internal carotid artery is suddenly blocked.

165. Cerebral arteries

(a) Anterior and middle cerebral arteries arise from the internal carotid artery.

(b) The visual areas are supplied mainly by the posterior cerebral artery.

(c) Somatic motor and somatic sensory areas are supplied exclusively by the anterior cerebral artery.

(d) Speech and auditory areas lie in the territory of the middle cerebral artery.

(e) Arterial twigs entering the brain substance are end arteries.

166. Central arteries of the cerebrum

(a) These are end arteries and supply the basal nuclei and deeper parts of the cerebral white matter.

(b) These are divisible into four groups; anterolateral, anteromedial, posterolateral and posteromedial.

(c) The anterolateral (striate) arteries are divided into medial and lateral groups in relation to the lentiform nucleus.

(d) Heubner's artery (recurrent branch of anterior cerebral artery) supplies anterior part of the caudate nucleus.

(e) The Charcot's artery (of cerebral haemorrhage), most commonly involved in cerebrovascular accidents, is usually the largest of all medial striate central arteries.

167. Arterial supply of cerebellum and brainstem

(a) The arterial supply of cerebellum is derived from basilar and vertebral arteries.

(b) The midbrain derives its arterial supply from the basilar artery.

(c) The pons is mainly supplied by basilar artery through its 3 sets of branches; paramedian, short circumferential and long circumferential.

(d) The medulla oblongata receives its supply largely from the vertebral arteries.

(e) Thrombosis in the posterior inferior cerebellar artery is responsible for the medial medullary syndrome.

168. Base of the brain

(a) Anterior perforated substance is located on each side of the optic chiasma.

(b) Optic chiasma and tracts, crura cerebri, and pons form the boundaries of the interpeduncular fossa.

(c) Occulomotor nerve, posterior perforated substance, mamillary bodies and tuber cinereum are the structures lying in the interpeduncular fossa.

(d) V, VII, VIII, IX, X cranial nerves and cranial root of the XI cranial nerve are attached on the ventral aspect of brainstem.

(e) The IV cranial (trochlear) is the only nerve which emerges from the dorsal aspect of the brainstem and winds round the midbrain to appear on the base of the brain.

169. Midbrain–I

(a) It is the smallest segment of the brainstem.

(b) It is marked posteriorly by four rounded swellings (superior and inferior pairs of colliculi) called corpora quadrigemina.

(c) Its superior and inferior colliculi act as auditory and visual reflex centres, respectively.

(d) It consists of the two crura cerebri anteriorly.

(e) A median white ridge, extending from the groove between its inferior colliculi to the superior medullary velum, is called frenulum veli.

170. Midbrain–II

(a) Its narrow tubular cavity (cerebral aqueduct) connects the 3rd ventricle above with the 4th ventricle below.

(b) Its cross-sections at the level of superior colliculi can be recognized by the presence of red nucleus, inferior brachium and pretectal nucleus.

(c) The nuclei of III and IV cranial nerves are located at the levels of superior and inferior colliculi, respectively.

(d) Its two cerebral peduncles lie anterior to its cerebral aqueduct.

(e) The neurons of the substantia nigra are characterized by the presence of neuromelanin pigments and production of the acetylcholine.

171. Pons–I

(a) It is situated ventral to cerebellum, and in between midbrain and medulla oblongata.

(b) Its ventral surface is marked by a shallow median groove, called the sulcus basilaris, which lodges the basilar artery.

(c) Its lesion involving the principal sensory nucleus of V cranial nerve will cause anaesthesia to light touch over the trigeminal distribution, with preservation of pain and temperature sensibilities.

(d) The emergence of the facial nerve demarcates its junction with the middle cerebellar peduncle.

(e) Its dorsal surface contributes to upper half of the floor of the 4th ventricle.

172. Pons–II

(a) Its ventral (basilar) part shows continuity with the crura cerebri of midbrain, above and with the pyramids of medulla, below.

(b) The nuclei scattered in its ventral part (nuclei pontis) receive fibres descending from the entire cerebral cortex.

(c) All the four lemnisci (lateral, spinal, trigeminal and medial) ascend through it.

(d) The motor and the main sensory nuclei of the trigeminal nerve, and superior medullary velum are the features exclusively observed in the cross-sections through its lower part.

(e) Fibres arising from the facial nucleus run backwards, loop around the abducent nucleus and then course forwards to emerge on the ventral aspect of the brainstem.

173. Medulla oblongata–I

(a) It extends from the lower border of pons to a plane passing just above the 1st pair of cervical nerves.

(b) Its upper (open) part forms the lower part of the floor of the 4th ventricle.

(c) In its upper part, the anterior median fissure is obliterated by the interdigitations of bundles of fibres crossing obliquely, called the decussation of the pyramids.

(d) It is also called the bulb, a term often used in some clinical conditions, e.g. bulbar paralysis.

(e) Its anterolateral sulcus is marked by the attachments of rootlets of hypoglossal nerve.

174. Medulla oblongata–II

(a) The pyramidal tract produces a bulging anteriorly by the side of the midline.

(b) Spinocerebellar tracts are located close to its surface.

(c) Vestibular, cochlear and olivary nuclei, and the inferior cerebellar peduncles are the features specifically observed in cross-sections of its upper part.

(d) Internal arcuate fibres and their crossings (sensory decussation) are seen only in cross-sections of its middle portion.

(e) Its lower part is characterized by the pyramidal decussation which leads to the formation of anterior corticospinal tracts.

175. Cerebellum–I

(a) It lies in the posterior cranial fossa below the tentorium cerebelli.

(b) It is divided by the two deep fissures (primary and posterolateral) into three lobes; anterior, middle and flocculonodular.

(c) Its median part, sandwiched between two cerebellar hemispheres, is called vermis.

(d) Its superior surface is supplied by two superior cerebellar arteries while its inferior surface receives its blood supply from a single inferior cerebellar artery.

(e) It is connected anteriorly with the midbrain, pons and medulla by the superior, middle and inferior cerebellar peduncles, respectively.

176. Cerebellum–II

(a) The dentate, emboliform, fastigial and globose (d, e, f, g) nuclei are located deeply in its white matter.

(b) The mossy (spinocerebellar) and climbing (olivocerebellar) fibres synapse with its Purkinje cells directly and indirectly (via granular cells), respectively.

(c) The superior cerebellar peduncle is predominantly efferent, whereas the other two (middle and inferior) cerebellar peduncles are afferent in nature.

(d) Its most primitive part, called archicerebellum, consists of flocculonodular lobe and lingula.

(e) It is concerned with accurate coordination of movements of the muscles.

177. Fourth ventricle

(a) It is the diamond-shaped cavity of pons and upper medulla.

(b) Its each lateral wall is formed by two peduncles (superior and inferior cerebellar) and two tubercles (gracile and cuneate).

(c) It communicates with the subarachnoid space through two lateral apertures (of Luschka) and one median aperture (of Magendie).

(d) Each half of its floor is divided by the sulcus limitans into a lateral part, vestibular area, and a medial part, medial eminence.

(e) The medial eminence is marked below the striae medullares by a rounded swelling, called facial colliculus.

178. Cerebrum–I

(a) Each cerebral hemisphere is divided into four lobes; frontal, parietal, temporal and occipital.

(b) Somatic sensory (areas 3, 1, 2) and somatic motor (area 4) areas are located in the precentral and postcentral gyri, respectively.

(c) Motor speech area of Broca (areas 44, 45) lies in the inferior frontal gyrus.

(d) First acoustic area (area 41) largely corresponds with the anterior transverse temporal gyrus.

(e) Both the walls of calcarine sulcus together correspond with first visual area (area 17), called striate cortex.

179. Cerebrum–II

(a) Its white matter contains three types of fibres; association, commissural and projection.

(b) The corpus callosum constitutes the most conspicuous example of the commissural fibres.

(c) The projection fibres may be either afferent (corticopetal) or efferent (corticofugal) in nature.

(d) The short and long association fibres connect the ipsilateral adjoining gyri and the distant parts of cortex, respectively.

(e) The internal capsule is a collection of association fibres.

180. Third ventricle

(a) It is the narrow median cavity of mesencephalon.

(b) Its each lateral wall is marked by the hypothalamic sulcus, separating thalamus from hypothalamus.

(c) Its roof is contributed by the tela choroidea and the ependyma adherent to it.

(d) It communicates with the lateral ventricles through interventricular foramen (of Monro).

(e) Its floor is contributed by the hypothalamus.

181. Lateral ventricle

(a) It is the cavity of telencephalic vesicle.

(b) The floor of its central part is contributed by caudate nucleus and stria terminalis, which also continue in the roof of its inferior horn.

(c) The choroid fissure for its choroid plexus does not extend into its anterior and posterior horns.

(d) Its anterior horn and central part are roofed by the corpus callosum.

(e) The collateral eminence of its posterior horn and the calcar avis of its inferior horn are produced by the collateral and calcarine sulci, respectively.

182. Limbic system

(a) Hippocampal formation and piriform lobe are the two important components of the limbic system.

(b) It is mainly concerned with the integration of olfactory, visceral and somatic impulses.

(c) It has nothing to do with the memories.

(d) It controls the activities necessary for survival of the species.

(e) Amygdaloid body, fornix and stria terminalis are included in the limbic system.

183. Diencephalon

(a) Thalamus is a large ovoid grey mass in the lateral wall of the third ventricle.

(b) Functionally, the thalamus is considered to be a great sensory relay station for the cerebral cortex.

(c) Medial and lateral geniculate bodies, together constituting the metathalamus, are relay stations in auditory and visual pathways, respectively.

(d) Pineal body and habenula together form the subthalamus.

(e) Hypothalamus, situated below the anterior part of the thalamus, regulates the endocrine, autonomic and behavioural activities.

184. Basal ganglia

(a) The basal ganglia consist of corpus striatum (caudate and lentiform nuclei), claustrum and amygdaloid complex.

(b) Phylogenetically the caudate nucleus, and putamen of the lentiform nucleus constitute the paleostriatum, whereas the globus pallidus forms the neostriatum.

(c) The basal ganglia are involved in the planning and programming of the movements.

(d) Corpus striatum receives afferents from the cerebral cortex, thalamus and substantia nigra.

(e) Afferents from the substantia nigra carry dopamine, the deficiency of which leads to the Parkinsonism.

185. Ascending tracts

(a) The 2nd order neurons in the posterior column-medial lemniscus pathway are situated in the gracile and cuneate nuclei.

(b) The lateral spinothalamic tract, carrying pain and temperature sensations, is usually spared in the syringomyelia.

(c) Anterior and posterior spinocerebellar tracts reach the cerebellum through superior and inferior cerebellar peduncles, respectively.

(d) Perception of pain is possible at the level of thalamus.

(e) Sensations of touch are carried through both anterior spinothalamic and posterior column-medial lemniscus pathways.

186. Descending tracts

(a) They consist of two components, pyramidal and extrapyramidal.

(b) Pyramidal tract is a three neuron pathway.

(c) Upper motor neuron paralysis results into rigidity and minimal wasting of the muscles.

(d) Pyramidal tract is facilitatory to the flexors whereas inhibitory to the extensors.

(e) The cerebral cortex controls the cerebellar activity through the corticoponto-cerebellar pathway.

187. Internal capsule

(a) It is the collection of projection fibres between lentiform nucleus medially, and thalamus and caudate nucleus laterally.

(b) It is continuous above and below with the corona radiata and crus cerebri, respectively.

(c) It consists of anterior limb, genu, posterior limb, and retrolentiform and sublentiform parts.

(d) Its genu and posterior limb are occupied by corticonuclear and corticospinal fibres, respectively.

(e) Its blood supply is derived mostly from the striate branches of middle cerebral and anterior choroidal arteries.

188. Visual pathway

(a) The optic nerve is the collection of axons of the ganglion cells of the retina.

(b) The optic nerve fibres derived from temporal half of the retina cross at optic chiasma to enter the opposite optic tract.

(c) Ipsilateral fibres in optic tract end in laminae 2, 3, 5 while the contralateral ones terminate in laminae 1, 4, 6 of the lateral geniculate body.

(d) The fibres emerging from the lateral geniculate body fan out to form the optic radiation, which ends in the visual cortex.

(e) A point to point relationship is maintained between retina, lateral geniculate body and visual cortex.

189. Auditory pathway

(a) The cochlear nerve consists of axons of the neurons of the spiral ganglion.

(b) The ventral and dorsal cochlear nuclei are placed on the corresponding aspect of the superior cerebellar peduncle.

(c) The fibres derived from cochlear and superior olivary nuclei, and nucleus of the trapezoid body ascend up and constitute the lateral lemniscus.

(d) Due to multiple crossings in the auditory pathway, its unilateral involvement in brain lesions usually fails to cause total deafness.

(e) The auditory radiation runs through the sublentiform part of the internal capsule to end in the auditory cortex.

HEAD AND NECK

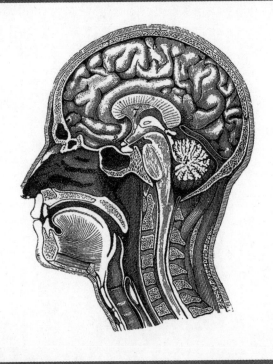

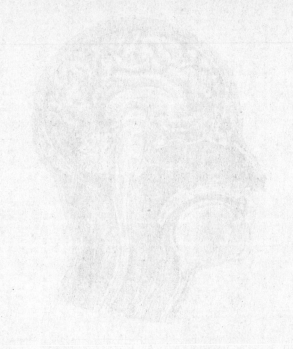

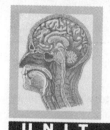

HEAD AND NECK

Find out incorrect statement in each set.

190. Typical (3rd to 6th) cervical vertebrae

(a) These are smallest movable vertebrae.

(b) These are identified by foramina transversaria.

(c) Their superior and inferior vertebral notches are equal in depth.

(d) Most of their transverse processes (ventral root, anterior tubercle, intertubercular lamella, posterior tubercle and lateral part of dorsal root) constitute the homologous of ribs while medial parts of their dorsal roots represent the true transverse processes.

(e) Carotid tubercle is large anterior tubercle of transverse process of 5th cervical vertebra against which the internal carotid artery can be effectively compressed.

191. Atypical (1st, 2nd and 7th) cervical vertebrae

(a) 1st cervical vertebra (atlas) supports the globe of the head and differs from other vertebrae in lacking a body.

(b) Anterior arch of atlas is formed by hypochordal bow, which is represented in thorax by the intermediate strand of the triradiate ligament of the head of the rib.

(c) Destruction of transverse ligament of atlas (commonly due to tuberculosis) leads to forward dislocation of atlas and consequent crushing of spinal cord between posterior arch and dens.

81

(d) Transverse process of the 7th cervical vertebra is most massive and hence its name, vertebra prominens.

(e) The axis vertebra provides the pivot around which the atlas and the head both rotate.

192. Skull

(a) Anterior fontanelle lies at the junction of sagittal, frontal and coronal sutures and is closed usually by 18 months.

(b) The skull is described to be brachy-, meso- and dolicho-cephalic when the cranial index (100 × maximal breadth/maximal length) is less than 75, from 75 to 80 and more than 80, respectively.

(c) Pterion (a small area enclosing 4 bones: frontal, parietal, temporal and sphenoid) is related to the anterior branch of middle meningeal artery.

(d) The bones in the base of skull are mostly cartilaginous while those in the vault are mainly membranous in origin.

(e) Reid's base line and Frankfurt's horizontal plane both pass anteriorly through the infraorbital margin while posteriorly they pass through the central point and upper margin of the external acoustic meatus, respectively.

193. Suture

(a) Sutural ligament between the bones consists of 5 layers— 2 cambial, 2 capsular and 1 middle.

(b) It is limited to skull.

(c) It is the mesenchymatous sheet which remains unossified during the development.

(d) The lambdoid suture is mostly denticulate in type.

(e) Sutural ligament never ossifies.

194. Auricle

(a) Auricular tubercle (of Darwin) is a swelling in helix and represents the primitive apex of pinna in lower animals.

(b) The lobule is the most dependent part of the auricle and is devoid of cartilage.

(c) The skin is loosely attached with its elastic fibrocartilaginous framework and therefore inflammatory conditions of the auricle are not very painful.

(d) The auricular muscles are supplied by the temporal and posterior auricular branches of facial nerve.

(e) Its sensory supply is derived from auriculotemporal, lesser occipital and great auricular nerves and auricular branch of the vagus nerve.

195. External nose

(a) Its bony framework consists of nasal bones, nasal parts of the frontal bones and frontal processes of the maxillae.

(b) Its cartilaginous support is derived from septal, lateral and alar (major and minor) nasal cartilages.

(c) Skin over the apex and alae is thickened, more firmly adherent and contains large sebaceous glands.

(d) Fracture of nasal bones, usually horizontal and in the upper one-third, is a common occurrence.

(e) Irritation of nostril leads to reflex lacrimation due to a common source of innervation, i.e. ophthalmic nerve.

196. Orbital opening

(a) Supraorbital margin, contributed entirely by the frontal bone, is rounded in its medial one-third and sharp in its lateral two-thirds.

(b) Its lateral margin is entirely formed by the frontal bone.

(c) The upper and lower parts of its medial margin are formed by frontal bone and frontal process of the maxilla, respectively.

(d) Infraorbital margin is contributed by the zygomatic bone, laterally and the maxilla, medially.

(e) Le Fort III is a horizontal fracture involving upper part of orbital opening and superior orbital fissure.

197. Anterior nasal aperture

(a) It is rounded in shape.

(b) It is bounded below by the maxillae and above by the nasal bones.

(c) Anterior ethmoidal nerve continues through an aperture at the lower margin of nasal bone as external nasal nerve.

(d) Its lower margin along with the adjacent lateral margin constitutes the nasal notch.

(e) Le Fort I is a horizontal fracture of the maxillae just above the alveolar process and it passes through the lower part of the nasal aperture.

198. Orbital cavity

(a) Orbital plates of the frontal and lesser wings of the sphenoid are the bones forming its roof.

(b) Its floor is contributed mainly by maxilla and also by zygomatic and palatine bones.

(c) Its lateral wall is formed by greater wing of sphenoid and frontal process of zygomatic bone.

(d) Bones lying in its medial wall from before backwards are— frontal process of maxilla, lacrimal, ethmoid (lamina papyracea) and body of sphenoid.

(e) Interior of the orbit is most conveniently approached from medial side as the eyeball is farthest from its medial wall.

199. External acoustic meatus (medial bony part)

(a) Major contribution to its boundary is derived from squamous part of temporal bone.

(b) Suprameatal (Macewen's) triangle, an area above and behind the meatus, is marked by suprameatal spine of Henle and forms the lateral wall of mastoid antrum which is 1.2 cm deep to the surface in adults.

(c) It contributes one-third, half and two-thirds of the total length (24 mm) of external acoustic meatus in infants, 5 years old children and adults, respectively.

(d) Narrowest part (isthmus) of external acoustic meatus is located in the bony part and lies 2 cm deep to the floor of concha.

200. Styloid process

(a) It is a 2.5 cm long projection from inferior surface of temporal bone and is divisible into upper (tympanohyal) and lower (stylohyal) parts.

(b) It develops from the cartilage (Meckel's) of 1st pharyngeal (mandibular) arch.

(c) It provides attachment to 3 muscles—stylohyoid, stylo-pharyngeus and styloglossus (supplied by VII, IX and XII cranial nerves, respectively) and two ligaments—stylohyoid and stylomandibular.

(d) It is related laterally to the parotid (facial nerve, retro-mandibular vein and external carotid artery being buried in the gland) and medially to the internal jugular vein.

(e) A very long styloid process, which develops due to ossification of stylohyoid ligament in continuity, can be felt at the side of pharynx behind the tonsil.

201. Superior orbital fissure

(a) It is a linear gap bounded above, below and medially by lesser and greater wings and body of sphenoid bone, respectively.

(b) Common tendinous ring (of Zinn) for extrinsic muscles of eyeball divides it into lateral, intermediate and medial parts.

(c) Lateral narrow part provides passage to lacrimal, frontal and trochlear (LFT) nerves from lateral to medial side.

(d) Oculomotor, abducent and maxillary nerves enter the orbit through the tendinous ring.

(e) Superior and inferior ophthalmic veins generally pass through its lateral and medial parts, respectively.

202. Scalp–I

(a) Skin (S), connective tissue (C), aponeurosis (A), loose areolar tissue (L) and pericranium (P) constitute the five layers of scalp, of which the superficial three layers fuse together to form the first surgical layer.

(b) Its skin is relatively less sensitive and more prone to sebaceous cysts.

(c) Damage to its second layer leads to profuse bleeding because the walls of the traversing blood vessels are anchored to the surrounding dense connective tissue.

(d) In case of haemorrhage in fourth layer, the blood usually extends laterally and posteriorly only up to zygomatic arch and highest nuchal line, respectively but anteriorly, it may reach the eyelids (black eye).

(e) The swelling produced by cephalohematoma (collection of blood deep to pericranium) lies across the sutures.

203. Scalp–II

(a) It receives profuse arterial supply from external carotid only.

(b) The veins (named after the arteries) from its anterior, middle and posterior parts drain into internal jugular vein, subclavian vein and suboccipital venous plexus, respectively.

(c) The lymphatics from its anterior, middle and posterior parts drain into preauricular (parotid), postauricular (mastoid) and occipital lymph nodes, respectively.

(d) Quick healing of its wounds is due to the rich vascularity of the region.

(e) Emissary veins connect extracranial veins with intracranial venous sinuses and therefore may transmit the infections from exterior to interior of cranium.

204. Scalp–III

(a) Its anterior part (up to interauricular line) is supplied by branches of ophthalmic (supratrochlear and supraorbital), maxillary (zygomaticotemporal) and mandibular (auriculotemporal) divisions of trigeminal nerve.

(b) Its posterior part is innervated by branches of ventral (great auricular–C_2, C_3 and lesser occipital–C_2) and dorsal (greater occipital–C_2 and third occipital–C_3) rami.

(c) Facial nerve (temporal and posterior auricular branches) supplies occipitofrontalis and auricular muscles.

(d) Its sympathetic twigs are derived from middle cervical ganglion.

(e) Its inflammatory conditions are very painful due to unyielding nature of dense connective tissue layer.

205. Facial muscles

(a) Embryologically these muscles belong to 1st pharyngeal (mandibular) arch.

(b) These are primarily sphincters or dilators of the facial apertures while the facial expressions are produced secondarily as the side effects of their primary actions.

(c) Majority of these muscles regulate the oral orifice and two-thirds of them constitute the modiolar muscles (cruciate and transverse) on account of their attachment to the modiolus.

(d) Modiolus, a fibromuscular knot lying 1 cm lateral to angle of mouth opposite the upper 2nd premolar tooth, forms an important landmark for prosthetic dentistry.

(e) All these muscles are supplied by facial nerve which in Bell's palsy becomes oedematous in the rigid facial canal.

206. Deep cervical fascia

(a) It consists of investing, prevertebral and pretracheal laminae and carotid sheath.

(b) The investing lamina extends from mandibular base and superior nuchal line above to the outer border of 1st rib below.

(c) The pretracheal lamina encloses thyroid gland on account of which the gland moves up and down during swallowing.

(d) Its prevertebral lamina extends over anterior and lateral vertebral muscles from cranial base to 3rd thoracic vertebra.

(e) Its carotid sheath encloses common and internal carotid arteries, internal jugular vein, vagus nerve and ansa cervicalis.

207. Posterior triangle–I

(a) Its anterior and posterior boundaries and base are formed by sternomastoid, trapezius and middle 3rd of clavicle, respectively.

(b) Its roof is contributed by investing lamina of cervical fascia.

(c) Its floor is mainly formed by semispinalis capitis, levator scapulae and scalenus medius.

(d) It is divided into upper occipital and lower subclavian triangles by the inferior belly of omohyoid.

(e) Nerves to levator scapulae, rhomboids, serratus anterior and diaphragm run over its floor deep to prevertebral lamina.

208. Posterior triangle–II

(a) It is divided into upper 'carefree area' and lower 'danger area' by spinal accessory nerve which passes from midpoint of sternomastoid's posterior border to trapezius (5 cm above clavicle).

(b) Cutaneous nerves appearing in it are greater occipital, great auricular, transverse cervical and supraclavicular.

(c) It is traversed by subclavian, transverse cervical, suprascapular and occipital arteries.

(d) Local anaesthetic is injected into its upper and lower parts for cervical and brachial plexus block, respectively.

(e) Irritation of spinal accessory nerve (due to enlarged lymph nodes) leads to spasm of sternomastoid, also called as acute torticollis.

209. External jugular vein

(a) It is formed at the lower end of parotid gland by the union of superficial temporal and maxillary veins.

(b) It descends superficially over sternomastoid and pierces the investing lamina of cervical fascia in the subclavian triangle to join the subclavian vein.

(c) It has two incomplete valves (one at the entrance into subclavian vein and another 4 cm above clavicle) incompetent to prevent regurgitation.

(d) Its size is inversely proportional to other veins in the neck.

(e) Its laceration where it pierces the investing lamina may lead to venous air embolism.

210. Scalenus anterior

(a) Its fibres converge from the anterior tubercles of transverse processes of typical cervical vertebrae to scalene tubercle and a ridge anterior to the groove for subclavian artery on the 1st rib.

(b) It is innervated by ventral rami of all the cervical nerves.

(c) Acting from below it bends the neck anterolaterally, while acting from above it raises the first rib.

(d) Phrenic nerve descends on its anterior surface deep to prevertebral lamina.

(e) In about 70% of patients, the neurological symptoms of cervical rib syndrome are relieved by incising it near its insertion (scalenotomy).

211. Subclavian artery

(a) It extends either from arch of aorta (on left side) or brachiocephalic trunk (on right side) to outer border of 1st rib.

(b) It is represented on the surface by an arch with convexity upwards, a little above the medial half of the clavicle.

(c) Its 1st, 2nd and 3rd parts lie proximal, deep and distal to scalenus anterior, respectively.

(d) Most of its branches (vertebral, internal thoracic, thyrocervical and costocervical) spring from the 3rd part while dorsal scapular artery arises usually from its 1st part.

(e) Its 3rd part, being easily accessible, can be compressed against 1st rib in the anteroinferior angle of posterior triangle in cases of traumatic haemorrhage.

212. Brachial plexus–I

(a) It is formed by the dorsal rami of cervical 5, 6, 7 and 8 and thoracic 1 spinal segments.

(b) Upper two (C_5, C_6) and lower two (C_8, T_1) roots unite to form upper and lower trunks respectively while the central root (C_7) continues as middle trunk.

(c) Only its roots and trunks lie in the neck.

(d) For brachial block, the needle is injected just above the midpoint of clavicle and directed below and medially to avoid the subclavian artery.

(e) Klumpke's paralysis (lower brachial lesion) leads to 'claw hand' deformity.

213. Brachial plexus–II

(a) Meeting point of two roots, two divisions and two branches (nerve to subclavius and suprascapular nerve) of the upper trunk is called as Erb's point.

(b) Dorsal scapular nerve springs from its highest root (C_5) to supply levator scapulae and rhomboids.

(c) Long thoracic nerve (of Bell) emerges from its upper three roots (C_5–C_7) and descends behind it.

(d) Its upper lesion (Erb-Duchenne or obstetrical paralysis) leads to 'wrist drop' deformity.

(e) Lesion of the long thoracic nerve results into 'winging' of scapula (undue prominence of medial border and inferior angle).

214. Trapezius

(a) Its fibres converge from skull, ligamentum nuchae, all thoracic spines and supraspinous ligaments to the pectoral girdle.

(b) Its motor supply comes from spinal accessory nerve while its proprioceptive fibres are derived from ventral rami of cervical 3 and 4.

(c) It is named as trapezius because it forms a trapezium (an irregular four-sided figure) along with its counterpart.

(d) Its upper and lower fibres along with lower four digitations of serratus anterior produce lateral rotation of scapula during abduction of arm.

(e) The trapezius myocutaneous flap is based on deep cervical artery and can be used to cover the defects of neck, face and scalp.

215. Thoracolumbar or lumbar fascia

(a) It covers the deep muscles of back of the trunk.

(b) It is trilaminar in the lumbar region and encloses quadratus lumborum and erector spinae in its anterior and posterior compartments, respectively.

(c) It is thin in the thoracic region and continues with its middle lamina in the lumbar region, below and investing lamina of the deep cervical fascia, above.

(d) Lateral arcuate ligament is the thickening (extending from transverse process of L_1 to rib 12) of its anterior lamina.

(e) Suppuration may, for some time, remain limited within the compartments of its laminae in the lumbar region.

216. Suboccipital triangle

(a) Its boundaries are formed by rectus capitis posterior major and minor and obliquus capitis superior.

(b) Posterior arch of atlas and posterior atlanto-occipital membrane lie in its floor.

(c) Semispinalis capitis and longissimus capitis form the medial and lateral parts of its roof, respectively.

(d) Its main contents are: Vertebral artery (3rd part), suboccipital nerve (C_1 dorsal ramus) and suboccipital venous plexus.

(e) Prolonged turning of head may lead to dizziness in cases of arteriosclerosed vertebral artery.

217. Facial artery–I

(a) It originates, in majority, from front of external carotid artery just above greater cornu of hyoid but in 43% cases it appears in common with lingual artery as linguo-facial trunk.

(b) It runs a very sinuous course in the neck (cervical part) as well as in face (facial part) to adapt to the movements in pharynx and face.

(c) Its cervical part is closely applied to the inferior aspect of submandibular gland where it arches over the posterior belly of digastric and stylohyoid muscle.

(d) Its cervical part gives off ascending palatine, tonsillar, glandular and submental arteries.

(e) It is vulnerable during surgical resection of submandibular gland.

218. Facial artery–II

(a) It enters the face at the anteroinferior angle of masseter and ends at the medial angle of eye.

(b) It runs posterior to facial vein and traverses a cleft in the modiolus.

(c) Superior and inferior labial and lateral nasal arteries are its branches in the face.

(d) Anaesthetists often palpate it against the mandibular base for pulse monitoring.

(e) Rich vascularity of the face accounts for profuse bleeding of the wounds on the one hand and quick healing of the same on the other.

219. Facial vein

(a) It is a valveless vein formed by the union of supraorbital and supratrochlear veins at the medial canthus of eye.

(b) It lies behind the facial artery and is less tortuous than the latter.

(c) It unites with anterior division of retromandibular vein to form common facial vein which enters the internal jugular vein.

(d) It communicates with cavernous sinus through ophthalmic veins and through deep facial vein via pterygoid venous plexus and emissary vein.

(e) 'Danger area' of face is a triangular area between angles of mouth and chin.

220. Cutaneous nerves of face

(a) Area of skin derived from frontonasal prominence is supplied by lacrimal, supraorbital, supratrochlear, infratrochlear and external nasal branches of ophthalmic nerve.

(b) Zygomaticotemporal, zygomaticofacial and infraorbital branches of maxillary nerve innervate the skin of maxillary prominence.

(c) The skin derived from the mandibular prominence is supplied by auriculotemporal, great auricular and mental branches of mandibular nerve.

(d) Postganglionic sympathetic fibres to the facial skin are derived from superior cervical ganglion.

(e) Retrogasserian neurotomy (i.e. root sectioning) results into permanent relief from pain of trigeminal neuralgia.

221. Eyelid

(a) It consists of skin, subcutaneous tissue, orbicularis oculi, tarsal plate and conjunctiva from anterior to posterior.

(b) Tarsal (Meibomian) glands add oily secretion to the tears.

(c) There are no eyelashes in the medial 1/6th of its margin.

(d) Its medial and lateral parts are drained by preauricular and submandibular lymph nodes, respectively.

(e) Stye results from the inflammation of gland of Zeis, a modified sebaceous gland.

222. Lacrimal apparatus–I (lacrimal gland)

(a) It consists of a larger orbital and a smaller palpebral part, the latter being visible through conjunctiva when the lid is everted.

(b) All its ducts (about a dozen) traverse through its palpebral part and hence excision of merely this part amounts to the total removal.

(c) Conjunctiva does not dry up after removal of the main gland due to the presence of many small accessory glands.

(d) Its preganglionic fibres run from inferior salivatory nucleus to pterygopalatine ganglion through facial, greater superficial petrosal and nerve of pterygoid canal (Vidian nerve).

(e) Its postganglionic secretomotor fibres emerge from pterygopalatine ganglion and run through maxillary, zygomatic and lacrimal nerves.

223. Lacrimal apparatus–II

(a) The lacrimal fluid traverses through conjunctival sac and lacrimal canaliculi, sac and duct to drain ultimately into inferior meatus.

(b) The lengths of lacrimal canaliculi, sac and duct are about 10, 12 and 18 mm, respectively.

(c) The upper and lower ends of lacrimal duct are marked by mucosal folds named as valve of Krause and valve of Hasner, respectively.

(d) Lacrimal part of orbicularis oculi produces dilatation of lacrimal sac during blinking and helps in the drainage of lacrimal fluid.

(e) Lacrimal sac is innervated by supratrochlear nerve.

224. Cranial dura mater

(a) It consists of an outer meningeal and an inner endosteal layer.

(b) There are four dural folds, two vertical (falx cerebri and cerebelli) and two horizontal (tentorium cerebelli and diaphragma sellae) derived from its meningeal layer, to minimise the rotatory displacement of brain.

(c) Its major portion in the supratentorial compartment is innervated by ophthalmic division of trigeminal nerve.

(d) Its blood supply is derived from both the carotid (external and internal) arteries.

(e) For intractable trigeminal neuralgia, rhizotomy (sectioning of trigeminal sensory root) is preferably performed in Meckel's cave, an evagination of lower layer of tentorium cerebelli over apex of petrous bone.

225. Cranial fossae–I

(a) Ophthalmic artery and veins run together in the optic canal.

(b) III and VI cranial and nasociliary nerves pass through common tendinous ring while lacrimal, frontal and trochlear (LFT) nerves traverse the lateral part of superior orbital fissure.

(c) Maxillary and mandibular nerves run through foramen rotundum and ovale, respectively.

(d) Internal carotid artery traverses only the upper part of foramen lacerum.

(e) It is the brain (medulla oblongata) which passes through foramen magnum.

226. Cranial fossae–II

(a) Hypophyseal (pituitary) fossa is a depression on the superior surface of body of sphenoid between tuberculum sellae anteriorly and dorsum sellae posteriorly.

(b) Middle meningeal artery and nervus spinosus pass through foramen spinosum.

(c) Internal acoustic meatus is traversed by IX, X and XI cranial nerves along with labyrinthine artery.

(d) Hypoglossal canal is meant for the passage of XII cranial nerve and meningeal branch of ascending pharyngeal artery.

(e) Middle meningeal vessels (the veins probably more often) are commonly involved in cases of fracture of skull.

227. Internal carotid artery–I

(a) It is named as internal because of its relative position with external carotid artery.

(b) It arises from common carotid artery in the neck at the level of superior border of thyroid cartilage and terminates inside the cranium by dividing into anterior and middle cerebral arteries.

(c) It is divisible, for descriptive purposes, into cervical, petrous, cavernous and cerebral parts.

(d) The carotid sinus is a bulbous dilatation at the bifurcation of common carotid artery, mainly involving the origin of internal carotid.

(e) Its cervical part can easily be differentiated from external carotid artery during operative procedures because of being devoid of any branch.

228. Internal carotid artery–II

(a) Its petrous, cavernous and cerebral parts adopt a very tortuous course with 6 bends to dampen the pulsation and maintain a continuous flow of blood to the brain.

(b) The hypophyseal and meningeal branches originate from its petrous part.

(c) The branches appearing from its cavernous part are cavernous, hypophyseal and meningeal arteries.

(d) Its cerebral part provides ophthalmic, anterior and middle cerebral, posterior communicating and anterior choroid arteries.

(e) Pulsating exophthalmos is a sign of carotico-cavernous fistula which may result from the fracture of skull base.

229. Petrosal nerves

(a) Greater petrosal nerve carries preganglionic parasympathetic fibres from superior salivatory nucleus to pterygopalatine ganglion.

(b) Deep petrosal nerve arising from internal carotid sympathetic plexus joins the greater petrosal nerve to form the nerve of pterygoid canal (Vidian nerve).

(c) Lesser petrosal nerve carries preganglionic secretomotor fibres from superior salivatory nucleus to otic ganglion for parotid gland.

(d) External petrosal nerve is an inconstant nerve connecting middle meningeal sympathetic plexus with genicular ganglion.

(e) Traction of greater petrosal nerve during surgical intervention of trigeminal (Gasserian) ganglion may lead to facial palsy.

230. Cranial dural venous sinuses–I

(a) These differ from a typical vein in being non-expansile and deprived of valves.

(b) The cavernus, sphenoparietal, petrosal (superior and inferior), transverse and sigmoid are paired sinuses.

(c) Sagittal (superior and inferior), straight and occipital belong to the unpaired group of sinuses.

(d) All the dural sinuses ultimately drain into external jugular vein.

(e) Tear in the walls of the sinuses during fracture of skull leads to persistent bleeding.

231. Cranial dural venous sinuses–II (cavernous sinus)

(a) It is about 2 cm long and 1 cm wide and lies by the side of body of sphenoid between medial end of superior orbital fissure and apex of petrous temporal bone.

(b) Abducent nerve and internal carotid artery (along with its sympathetic plexus) traverse its cavity.

(c) Oculomotor, trochlear, ophthalmic and maxillary nerves run in its lateral wall.

(d) It receives afferents from nose and paranasal sinuses and drains through superior and inferior petrosal sinuses into sigmoid sinus and internal jugular vein, respectively.

(e) Cavernous sinus thrombosis produces ipsilateral exophthalmos which soon becomes bilateral because of intercavernous sinuses.

232. Cranial dural venous sinuses–III

(a) The posterior dilated end of inferior sagittal sinus is termed as the confluence of sinuses or torcular Herophili.

(b) Straight sinus is formed by the union of inferior sagittal sinus and great cerebral vein of Galen.

(c) Superior sagittal sinus generally continues with the transverse sinus of right side while straight sinus becomes continuous with the transverse sinus of left side.

(d) Occipital sinus is situated between the two layers of falx cerebelli.

(e) Sigmoid sinus may be damaged during mastoidectomy due to its close relationship with mastoid antrum.

233. Orbit–I (extraocular muscles)

(a) Its striated group includes four recti (superior, inferior, medial and lateral), two obliqui (superior and inferior) and superficial lamella of levator palpebrae superioris.

(b) Deep lamella of levator palpebrae superioris, inferior tarsal muscle and orbitalis constitute its non-striated muscles.

(c) Rectus and oblique muscles produce one or combination of following movements of eyeball—adduction, abduction, elevation, depression, intorsion and extorsion.

(d) All the striated muscles are supplied by oculomotor nerve while the non-striated muscles have sympathetic innervation.

(e) An attempt to use a paralyzed rectus or oblique muscle produces two images, a condition called double vision (diplopia).

234. Orbit–II (ophthalmic vessels)

(a) The ophthalmic artery, a branch of carotid syphon, enters the optic canal below and medial to optic nerve.

(b) The ophthalmic artery crosses above the intraorbital part of optic nerve from lateral to medial along with ophthalmic vein in front and nasociliary nerve behind.

(c) Veins accompanying the branches of ophthalmic artery and vorticose veins (4-5) join to form two ophthalmic veins (superior and inferior) which drain mainly into cavernous sinus.

(d) The orbit is characterized by the absence of lymphatics.

(e) Thrombosis or embolism of central artery of retina leads to sudden total blindness.

235. Orbit–III (nerves)

(a) The optic nerve after running a course inside the cranium (10 mm), optic canal (5 mm) and orbit (25 mm) joins the back of eyeball 3 mm medial to its posterior pole.

(b) The nerves closely related to its lateral wall, roof, medial wall and floor are lacrimal, frontal, nasociliary and infraorbital, respectively.

(c) About 8–10 short ciliary nerves, emerging from ciliary ganglion, carry postganglionic parasympathetic fibres for lacrimal gland, sympathetic fibres for blood vessels and sensory fibres for eyeball including cornea.

(d) Sympathetic fibres derived from cavernous plexus (cavernous part of internal carotid plexus) run through ophthalmic, nasociliary and long ciliary nerves to reach the dilator pupillae.

(e) Foster Kennedy syndrome is characterised by optic atrophy on one side and papilloedema on the other side and can result from frontal lobe tumour.

236. Anterior triangle of neck

(a) Its boundaries are formed by anterior midline, sternomastoid, mandibular base and a line between mandibular angle and mastoid.

(b) It is divided into 4 triangles (muscular, digastric, carotid and corresponding half of the submental) by two bellies of digastric and inferior belly of omohyoid.

(c) Spinal accessory nerve passes between the superficial (sterno-mastoid, sterno-occipital and cleido-occipital) and deep (cleidomastoid) parts of sternocleidomastoid.

(d) Inferior and middle constrictors, hyoglossus and thyrohyoid muscles constitute the floor of carotid triangle.

(e) Mylohyoid forms the floor of submental triangle bounded by anterior bellies of digastric and body of hyoid.

237. Prevertebral region

(a) The anterior vertebral muscles include two longus (colli and capitis) and two rectus capitis (anterior and lateralis).

(b) Ventral ramus of 1st cervical nerve appears between rectus capitis anterior and lateralis.

(c) Cervical part of sympathetic chain lies over pretracheal fascia which intervenes between it and anterior vertebral muscles.

(d) All the cervical ganglia (superior, middle and inferior) provide somatic, visceral and vascular branches.

(e) Cervical sympathetic chain lesion leads to Horner's syndrome, characterised by miosis, partial ptosis, enophthalmos and facial vasodilatation and anhydrosis.

238. Infrahyoid muscles

(a) Sternohyoid, omohyoid (superior and inferior bellies), sternothyroid and thyrohyoid are the infrahyoid muscles.

(b) These muscles are innervated by upper 3 cervical spinal segments via XII cranial nerve and ansa cervicalis.

(c) This group of muscles depresses the larynx or hyoid or fixes the hyoid during mandibular depression.

(d) The lower end of omohyoid is attached to scapula during foetal life and persists as such in adult life too.

(e) The tendinous intersections, occasionally present in sternohyoid, indicate the segmental origin of the muscle from paravertebral myotomes.

239. Preauricular region

(a) Masseter, the most superficial muscle of mastication, produces depression of mandible.

(b) From superficial to deep, facial nerve, retromandibular vein and external carotid artery lie in the parotid gland.

(c) Secretomotor fibres of parotid derived from inferior salivatory nucleus reach the gland through glossopharyngeal nerve, tympanic plexus, lesser petrosal nerve, otic ganglion and auriculotemporal nerve.

(d) Parotid duct, about 5 cm in length and 5 mm in width, opens in the vestibule opposite the upper 2nd molar tooth.

(e) Frey's syndrome, characterised by beads of perspiration and hyperaesthesia on face during salivation, results due to auriculotemporal nerve injury.

240. Facial nerve

(a) Its nuclei (motor, superior salivatory and tractus solitarius) are located in the lower pons.

(b) It has four bends, 1st at facial colliculus, 2nd at genicular ganglion, 3rd at aditus to antrum and 4th at stylomastoid foramen.

(c) Greater superficial petrosal (emerging from genicular ganglion) and chorda tympani (appearing 6 mm above the stylomastoid foramen) nerves belong absolutely to the nervus intermedius component.

(d) It is motor for 2nd branchial arch muscles, gustatory for anterior two-thirds of tongue and secretomotor for lacrimal gland, mouth cavity, nasal cavity, paranasal sinuses and nasopharynx.

(e) Its damage proximal to genicular ganglion leads to partial loss of function.

241. Temporal fossa

(a) It is bounded above by superior temporal line and below by zygomatic arch and infratemporal crest.

(b) The bones contributing to it are parietal, sphenoid, temporal and occipital.

(c) Skin, loose connective tissue, thin aponeurosis, temporal fascia, temporalis muscle and the pericranium are the layers lying superficial to deep in this region.

(d) Temporalis muscle extends from temporal fossa to coronoid process and causes mandibular elevation and retraction.

(e) It is a rare site for subepicranial hematoma as the pericranium is adherent to the bone here.

242. Infratemporal fossa–I

(a) It is located deep to mandibular ramus, below sphenoidal greater wing, lateral to pharynx behind maxillary body and in front of carotid sheath.

(b) Its contents are pterygoid muscles (medial and lateral), sphenomandibular ligament, maxillary artery, pterygoid venous plexus, mandibular nerve, otic ganglion and chorda tympani.

(c) The maxillary artery has 3 parts: mandibular, pterygoid and pterygopalatine.

(d) Medial aspect of mandibular neck is related to maxillary artery, maxillary vein and auriculotemporal nerve from above downwards.

(e) Pterygoid venous plexus could easily get punctured by the needle introduced to inject either alcohol into Gasserian ganglion or an anaesthetic solution to block the posterior superior alveolar nerve.

243. Infratemporal fossa–II (mandibular nerve)

(a) It is a mixed nerve formed by the union of a sensory and a motor root just beyond its exit through foramen ovale where it passes between lateral pterygoid and tensor palati.

(b) Its main trunk is located 4 cm from surface just posterior to mandibular neck.

(c) Nerve to medial pterygoid and the meningeal branch (nervus spinosus) emerge from the mandibular nerve before it splits into small anterior and large posterior trunks.

(d) All the branches of its anterior trunk are motor (for masseter, temporalis and lateral pterygoid muscles) except the buccal nerve which is sensory.

(e) Its posterior trunk, mainly sensory, divides into auriculotemporal, lingual and inferior alveolar nerves of which the last one also provides motor fibres (mylohyoid nerve) for mylohyoid and anterior belly of digastric.

244. Infratemporal fossa–III (otic ganglion)

(a) It is located between mandibular nerve (lateral), tensor palati (medial) and middle meningeal artery (posterior).

(b) Its communications with the nerve of pterygoid canal and chorda tympani explains an additional pathway through which gustatory fibres from presulcal area of tongue may reach the facial (genicular) ganglion without traversing the middle ear.

(c) Its secretomotor (parasympathetic) root for the parotid is formed by lesser petrosal nerve while its sympathetic root for parotid vasculature comes from the middle meningeal plexus.

(d) It receives an additional root from nerve to medial pterygoid for tensor tympani and palati.

(e) Its branches join the facial nerve to supply the parotid gland.

245. Temporomandibular joint

(a) It is a condylar type of synovial joint between temporal bone and mandible.

(b) Its articular disc has five parts from anterior to posterior: anterior extension, anterior band, middle zone, posterior band and bilaminar region.

(c) It is innervated by inferior alveolar and deep temporal nerves.

(d) Movements taking place at this joint are protraction and retraction, depression and elevation and side to side movement.

(e) Its anterior dislocation is commonest to occur.

246. Pterygopalatine fossa

(a) It is bounded by pterygoid process of sphenoid, palatine process of maxilla and perpendicular plate of palatine bone.

(b) Its main contents include maxillary nerve, pterygopalatine ganglion and 3rd part of maxillary artery.

(c) Ganglionic, posterior superior alveolar, zygomatic and infraorbital nerves are the branches arising from maxillary nerve in the fossa.

(d) The nerve of pterygoid canal (Vidian nerve) carries sympathetic and parasympathetic fibres while maxillary nerve provides sensory root to the pterygopalatine ganglion whose branches supply palate, nasal cavity, paranasal sinuses and nasopharynx.

(e) Pterygopalatine ganglion is also known as ganglion of hay fever which when very severe may warrant Vidian neurectomy.

247. Digastric

(a) It is composed of a bipennate posterior belly (attached to digastric notch of temporal bone) and an anterior belly (attached to digastric fossa at the anterior end of mandibular base).

(b) Its two bellies meet at an intermediate tendon which is held in position by a fibrous sling attached to the hyoid.

(c) Its anterior and posterior bellies are derived from the 2nd and 1st pharyngeal arches, respectively.

(d) Its anterior belly along with mylohyoid is innervated by the mylohyoid nerve while its posterior belly along with stylohyoid receives the nerve supply from the facial nerve.

(e) It assists the lateral pterygoid in mandibular depression.

248. Submandibular salivary gland

(a) It is a mixed type of salivary gland in which serous acini predominate.

(b) Its superficial and deep parts meet behind the posterior border of hyoglossus muscle.

(c) Stylomandibular ligament intervenes between it and the parotid gland.

(d) The submandibular (Wharton's) duct, about 5 cm long, opens at lingual papilla and is a common site for calculus.

(e) For surgical operations on this gland incision should be given at least one inch below the mandibular angle to save the mandibular branch of facial nerve.

249. Hyoglossus

(a) It is a quadrilateral muscle extending from hyoid (greater cornu and body) to the side of tongue where it lies between styloglossus (lateral) and inferior longitudinal muscle (medial).

(b) It is innervated by the hypoglossal nerve.

(c) It pulls the tongue backwards.

(d) From above downwards lie, lingual nerve, submandibular ganglion, deep part of submandibular gland and hypoglossal nerve superficial to it.

(e) Glossopharyngeal nerve and lingual blood vessels are located deep to it.

250. Sublingual salivary gland

(a) It is smallest of the main salivary glands and weighs about 3-4 grams.

(b) It lies in contact with sublingual fossa of mandible and produces sublingual mucosal fold.

(c) It has 8-20 excretory ducts most of which open separately on the summit of the sublingual fold while a few of them may join the submandibular duct.

(d) It is supplied by sublingual branch of the lingual artery and submental branch of the facial artery.

(e) Its innervation is derived from hypoglossal nerve and external carotid sympathetic plexus.

251. Thyroid gland

(a) It is an endocrine gland derived from thyroglossal duct and ultimobranchial body.

(b) The medial surface of its lobe is related to 2 tubes (trachea and oesophagus), 2 muscles (inferior constrictor and cricothyroid), 2 cartilages (thyroid and cricoid), 2 membranes (cricothyroid and cricotracheal) and 2 nerves (recurrent and external laryngeal).

(c) Pretracheal fascia provides a false capsule to it which is adherent to the cricoid by Berry's ligaments.

(d) Partial thyroidectomy is preferred by the surgeons to save the parathyroid glands and recurrent laryngeal nerves.

(e) Superior thyroid artery is ligated farther from gland while inferior thyroid artery is tied nearer to it to protect the external and recurrent laryngeal nerves, respectively.

252. Trachea

(a) It is a 10–11 cm long fibromuscular tube supported by cartilaginous rings and extends from 6th cervical vertebra to the intervertebral disc between 4th and 5th thoracic vertebrae.

(b) Its inner diameter is 3 mm in 1st year, then its diameter in mm is equal to the age in year till it attains the adult size (12 mm)

(c) Its cartilaginous rings are deficient anteriorly for trachealis muscle.

(d) Its arterial supply is derived from inferior thyroid and bronchial arteries.

(e) Tracheo-oesophageal fistula results from incomplete division of foregut into respiratory and digestive tubes.

253. Vertebral artery

(a) It emerges from the 3rd part of subclavian artery and ends by meeting its fellow of opposite side at the upper border of pons to form the basilar artery.

(b) Its 1st, 2nd, 3rd and 4th parts are located in the triangle of vertebral artery, upper 6 foramina transversaria, suboccipital triangle and cranium, respectively.

(c) Its 1st and 3rd parts are more elastic as these parts have greater mobility and lack any support.

(d) Its branches are grouped as cervical (spinal and muscular arteries) and cranial (meningeal, anterior and posterior spinal, posterior inferior cerebellar and medullary arteries).

(e) Thrombosis of posterior inferior cerebellar artery leads to lateral medullary (Wallenberg's) syndrome characterised by dysphonia, dysphagia and loss of pain and thermal sensibility on ipsilateral face and contralateral body.

254. External carotid artery

(a) It begins at the upper border of thyroid cartilage as one of the terminal branches of common carotid artery.

(b) It terminates just behind the mandibular neck into maxillary and superficial temporal arteries.

(c) Ascending pharyngeal artery arises from its medial aspect, occipital and posterior auricular arteries emerge from its posterior aspect and facial, lingual and superior thyroid arteries spring from its anterior aspect.

(d) In children, it is larger than internal carotid artery but in adults both are almost of equal size.

(e) Its ligation is preferably performed between the emergence of superior thyroid and lingual arteries.

255. Glossopharyngeal nerve

(a) It receives fibres from various nuclei which are sensory (spinal nucleus of trigeminal, tractus solitarius), motor (nucleus ambiguus) and secretomotor (inferior salivatory nucleus) in nature.

(b) It emerges through jugular foramen and then passes between external and internal carotid arteries to enter the pharyngeal part of the tongue.

(c) Its branches are tympanic, carotid, pharyngeal, muscular, tonsillar and lingual.

(d) Glossopharyngeal neuralgia is very rare as compared to trigeminal neuralgia.

(e) Its lingual branches receive general and taste sensations from posterior one-third of tongue excluding sulcus terminalis and vallate papillae.

256. Vagus nerve

(a) It receives sensory fibres from spinal nucleus of trigeminal nerve (general sensation from external acoustic meatus), dorsal nucleus (sensation from viscera) and solitarius nucleus (taste from epiglottis and vallecula).

(b) Its motor fibres originate in dorsal nucleus (for smooth visceral muscles), nucleus ambiguus (for skeletal muscles of pharynx and larynx) and inferior salivatory nucleus (secretomotor for visceral glands).

(c) It runs a vertical course in front of the groove between internal jugular vein and accompanying carotid artery (internal or common) in the carotid sheath.

(d) Its cervical part on each side gives rise to two cardiac branches, but only the left inferior branch goes to the superficial cardiac plexus while the rest contribute to the deep one.

(e) Injury to it or its nucleus leads to palpitation, tachycardia, slow respiration and feeling of suffocation.

257. Accessory nerve

(a) Its cranial root originates in both nucleus ambiguus as well as dorsal vagal nucleus.

(b) Its spinal root emerges from anterior grey column of upper five cervical spinal segments and ascends between ligamentum denticulatum and ventral spinal roots.

(c) Its cranial part (internal ramus) joins the vagus and is distributed mainly through pharyngeal and recurrent laryngeal branches of vagus to the striated muscles.

(d) Its spinal part (external ramus) constitutes motor supply of sternomastoid and trapezius.

(e) Its irritation due to cervical lymphadenitis may lead to torticollis.

258. Hypoglossal nerve

(a) Its somatic motor nucleus is located in the hypoglossal trigone in upper part of floor of 4th ventricle.

(b) It receives a communication from 1st cervical nerve at its exit from hypoglossal canal, and then it crosses the internal carotid, occipital, external carotid and lingual arteries to enter the tongue.

(c) Its C_1 fibres are distributed through the meningeal branch, descendens hypoglossi (for infrahyoid muscles) and nerve to thyrohyoid and geniohyoid.

(d) The fibres of hypoglossal nerve itself innervate all the intrinsic and extrinsic (except palatoglossus) muscles of tongue.

(e) Its complete division leads to ipsilateral lingual paralysis and atrophy.

259. Cervical sympathetic trunk

(a) Superior (3 cm long) and middle cervical ganglia lie at the level of first 2 cervical and 6th cervical vertebrae, respectively.

(b) Inferior cervical ganglion is often fused with the 1st thoracic ganglion to form cervicothoracic (stellate) ganglion (1 cm long).

(c) The superior, middle and inferior cervical ganglia give somatic branches to anterior primary rami of first two, next two and last four cervical spinal nerves, respectively.

(d) Its ganglia give rise to visceral branches to cardiac plexuses.

(e) The vascular branches of middle cervical ganglion form the plexuses around the subclavian and inferior thyroid arteries while those of superior and inferior ganglia form the plexuses around carotids and vertebral artery, respectively.

260. Internal jugular vein

(a) It begins at jugular fossa as continuation of sigmoid sinus and ends behind the medial end of clavicle by joining the subclavian vein.

(b) The vein is represented on the surface by a broad band from mandibular angle to sternal end of clavicle.

(c) Its immediate medial relation is the internal or common carotid artery.

(d) Its tributaries are inferior petrosal sinus and facial, lingual, pharyngeal, superior and middle thyroid veins.

(e) In Queckenstedt's test, manual compression of both the internal jugular veins just above the clavicles is followed by increased pressure of spinal CSF.

261. Cervical plexus

(a) It is formed by upper 3 cervical ventral rami.

(b) It is situated behind internal jugular vein and sterno-cleidomastoid and in front of scalenus medius and levator scapulae.

(c) It provides cutaneous nerves to part of scalp, front and lateral aspects of neck, upper part of front of thorax and shoulder.

(d) It supplies muscles through its communication with hypo-glossal nerve, named muscular branches (phrenic nerve and inferior root of ansa cervicalis) and unnamed muscular twigs.

(e) If an accessory phrenic nerve (C_5, via nerve to subclavius) exists, crushing of the main nerve in the neck will not produce complete diaphragmatic paralysis.

262. Scalene muscles

(a) Scalenus anterior extends from anterior tubercles of transverse processes of typical cervical vertebrae to scalene tubercle of 1st rib.

(b) Scalenus medius stretches from posterior tubercles of transverse processes of all cervical vertebrae to the 1st rib behind groove for subclavian artery.

(c) Scalenus posterior arises from posterior tubercles of upper cervical vertebral transverse processes and descends to get attached to the 2nd rib.

(d) These muscles are supplied by ventral rami of cervical 3 to 8 spinal segments.

(e) These muscles bend the neck ipsilaterally and also act as accessory respiratory muscles.

263. Root of neck

(a) It is defined as an area of the neck just above the inlet of thorax.

(b) Its midline contents are: trachea, oesophagus, both right and left recurrent laryngeal nerves and thoracic duct (vertical cervical part).

(c) On each side, it consists of lateral vertebral muscles, subclavian artery and its branches, subclavian and internal jugular veins, some nervous structures (phrenic, vagus, sympathetic chain and brachial plexus) and lower deep cervical lymph nodes.

(d) Scalene triangle (of vertebral artery) is bounded by 1st part of subclavian artery, scalenus anterior and longus colli.

(e) Stellate ganglion block is performed in this region to relieve the vascular spasm in face.

264. Lymphatics and lymph nodes of head and neck

(a) The external nose, cheek, upper lip and lateral part of lower lip are drained into submandibular lymph nodes.

(b) The central part of lower lip, floor of mouth and the tip of tongue are drained into submental nodes.

(c) Superficial lymphatics of head enter occipital, retroauricular (mastoid), parotid and buccal (facial) lymph nodes.

(d) Superficial lymphatics of neck drain into submandibular, submental, anterior cervical and superficial cervical lymph nodes.

(e) All the lymphatics of head and neck ultimately enter the deep cervical lymph nodes, whose efferents join to form subclavian trunk.

265. Joints of the neck

(a) Adjacent bodies of lower 6 cervical vertebrae form paired fibrous joints near lateral margins and unpaired secondary cartilaginous joints in the centre.

(b) Adjacent vertebral arches form synovial (called zygapophyseal) joints between articular processes and intervertebral syndesmoses between laminae and spines.

(c) Atlantoaxial joint includes a pair of zygapophyseal (plane type synovial) joints and an unpaired median pivot type of synovial joint between dens and anterior atlantal arch.

(d) Only 50% of rotation of head occurs at atlantoaxial joint.

(e) Atlanto-occipital joints are ellipsoid type of synovial joints and allow nodding as well as lateral flexion of head.

266. Mouth

(a) It is the first part of alimentary canal for taking food and talking.

(b) Suctorial pad of fat, a well-developed subcutaneous fatty mass in the cheek of infants, is very helpful in sucking process.

(c) It is divisible by teeth and gums into outer vestibule and inner oral cavity proper.

(d) The roof of oral cavity proper (hard palate) is innervated by the greater palatine and nasopalatine nerves while its floor is supplied by the inferior alveolar nerves.

(e) All the teeth at the age of 12 years are permanent.

267. Pharynx–I

(a) The fibres of superior constrictor interdigitate with those of buccinator along pterygomandibular raphe.

(b) The buccopharyngeal fascia covers the inner surfaces of the constrictors of pharynx.

(c) All the pharyngeal muscles are supplied by cranial accessory via vagus and pharyngeal plexus except crico- and stylo-pharyngeus, which are innervated by recurrent laryngeal and glossopharyngeal nerves, respectively.

(d) The sensory supply of the naso-, oro- and laryngopharynx is derived from pharyngeal branch of pterygopalatine ganglion, glossopharyngeal and laryngeal (recurrent and internal) nerves, respectively.

(e) Incoordination between cricopharyngeus and rest of the pharyngeal muscles may lead to the development of pharyngeal pouch.

268. Pharynx–II (nasopharynx)

(a) Its patency is maintained by thick membranous pharyngobasilar fascia.

(b) Opening of Eustachian tube is inverted 'J' shaped and lies just behind the posterior end of inferior nasal concha.

(c) Fossa of Rosenmuller (pharyngeal recess) is a narrow slit anterior to the opening of Eustachian tube.

(d) Pharyngeal, tubal, palatine and lingual tonsils together constitute the Waldeyer's ring.

(e) An enlarged pharyngeal tonsil is called adenoid.

269. Pharynx–III (oropharynx)

(a) The junction of naso- and oropharynx is marked by pharyngeal isthmus which is closed during swallowing to prevent the nasal regurgitation.

(b) The tonsil (palatine tonsil), a partially encapsulated lymphoid organ, is located in the triangular tonsillar sinus between palatoglossal and palatopharyngeal arches.

(c) Vallecula, a depression on each side, lies between median and lateral glosso-epiglottic folds.

(d) Posterior one-third of the dorsum of tongue belongs to oropharynx and is innervated by the lingual nerve for general sensation.

(e) Passavant's ridge, a muscular ridge produced by contraction of posterior fibres of palatopharyngeus at the level of pharyngeal isthmus, is very prominent in cases of cleft palate.

270. Pharynx–IV (laryngopharynx)

(a) Killian's dehiscence is the weakness in the pharyngeal wall in the region of thyropharyngeus above the vocal cords.

(b) Pharyngoepiglottic (lateral glossoepiglottic) folds separate the oropharynx from the laryngeal part of pharynx.

(c) Foreign body is commonly lodged in the piriform fossa which lies by the side of aryepiglottic fold.

(d) The lowest part of the pharynx lying behind the mucous membrane covered arytenoids and cricoid lamina is called hypopharynx.

(e) The laryngeal (internal and recurrent) nerves and laryngeal (superior and inferior) vessels anastomose freely in the wall of the pharynx before entering the larynx where there is a complete watershed for the nerves and vessels.

271. Soft palate

(a) It is a mobile muscular flap between oral cavity and oropharynx.

(b) Its musculature consists of tensor palati, levator palati, palatoglossus, palatopharyngeus and musculus uvulae.

(c) Its blood supply comes mainly from the ascending palatine (branch of facial) artery which first ascends to supply the pharynx and then descends to reach the soft palate.

(d) Its general as well as special sensory (taste) and the secreto-motor fibres are derived from the lesser palatine nerves.

(e) Its normal mobility confirms the integrity of the vagus which supplies its all the muscles except tensor palati, whose innervation comes from the mandibular nerve.

272. Auditory (eustachian) tube

(a) It is approximately 36 mm in length and forms an angle of 45° with the sagittal plane and an angle of 30° with the horizontal plane.

(b) Its medial two-thirds is osseous while its lateral one-third is cartilaginous.

(c) In younger children, it is relatively wider, shorter and more horizontal.

(d) Contraction of levator palati and salpingopharyngeus during deglutition and yawning causes opening of auditory tube.

(e) Its osteum, cartilaginous and bony parts are innervated by the pharyngeal branch of pterygopalatine ganglion, nervus spinosus and tympanic plexus, respectively.

273. Nose–I (nasal septum)

(a) The vomer, perpendicular plate of ethmoid and septal cartilage are the main components of its skeletal framework.

(b) Its anterosuperior part is innervated by the septal branch of anterior ethmoidal nerve while its posteroinferior part receives branches from the medial posterior superior nasal nerves and one of the latter constitutes the nasopalatine nerve.

(c) Veins from its anterior and posterior halves drain into ophthalmic vein and pterygoid venous plexus, respectively.

(d) Lymphatics from its anterior half enter the submandibular lymph nodes while those from its posterior half drain into the retropharyngeal or upper deep cervical lymph nodes.

(e) Four sets of arteries (anterior ethmoidal, superior labial branch of the facial, greater palatine and medial posterior superior nasal branches of the sphenopalatine) converge at Little's area, which is the commonest site of epistaxis.

274. Nose–II (nasal cavity)

(a) It is divisible into three parts: Vestibule, and olfactory and respiratory areas.

(b) Its lateral wall has 3 projections (superior, middle and inferior nasal conchae) and 4 depressions (3 meatuses lying inferior to the corresponding conchae and sphenoethmoidal recess situated superior to the superior concha) .

(c) Posterior half, anterosuperior and anteroinferior quadrants of its lateral wall, are innervated by pterygopalatine ganglion, anterior ethmoidal and anterior superior alveolar nerves, respectively.

(d) The anterior half of its lateral wall lies in the territory of internal carotid artery while the posterior half is supplied by external carotid artery.

(e) Anterior, middle and posterior parts of its lateral wall are drained by facial vein, pterygoid and pharyngeal venous plexuses, respectively.

275. Paranasal sinuses

(a) These are air filled spaces in the bones surrounding the nasal cavity.

(b) Majority of paranasal sinuses (maxillary, frontal and anterior and middle ethmoidal) drain into middle meatus while sphenoidal and posterior ethmoidal sinuses drain into sphenoethmoidal recess and superior meatus, respectively.

(c) Their important functions include–to lighten the skull, provide resonance to the voice, act as insulator, to warm and moisten the air and to push the mucus to nasal cavity.

(d) All these sinuses are present at birth in rudimentary form except the frontal one which may be absent and they rapidly enlarge during eruption of permanent teeth and after puberty.

(e) In antrostomy an artificial opening is made in the middle meatus to help the drainage of pus from the maxillary sinus.

276. Larynx–I (framework)

(a) It consists of 3 unpaired (thyroid, cricoid and epiglottis) and 3 paired (arytenoid, corniculate and cuneiform) cartilages.

(b) It has got extrinsic (thyrohyoid and cricotracheal membranes) and intrinsic (quadrate ligament and cricothyroid membrane) membranes or ligaments.

(c) Cricoarytenoid and cricothyroid joints are fibrous joints restricting movements of the laryngeal cartilages.

(d) Recurrent laryngeal nerve ascends deep to the lower margin of cricopharyngeus immediately behind the cricothyroid joint.

(e) Cricoarytenoid joints permit rotation or gliding of arytenoids to regulate the rima glottidis.

277. Larynx–II (interior)

(a) Inlet of larynx is directed forwards.

(b) Interior of the larynx above the vestibular folds is called the vestibule.

(c) The middle of interior of laryngeal cavity leads on each side into a sinus which provides a diverticulum called saccule of the larynx.

(d) Vocal cords form the watershed for the laryngeal blood vessels and lymphatics.

(e) Mucosa above the vocal cords is innervated by internal laryngeal branch of superior laryngeal nerve while the area below the vocal cords derives its nerve supply from the recurrent laryngeal nerve.

278. Larynx–III (intrinsic muscles)

(a) Thyroepiglottic and aryepiglottic muscles are responsible for regulating the inlet of the larynx.

(b) Lateral cricoarytenoids and interarytenoid are the muscles which open (abduct) the rima glottidis while posterior cricoarytenoid muscles cause its closure (adduction).

(c) Tension of the vocal cords is maintained by the cricothyroid and thyroarytenoid muscles.

(d) All the intrinsic muscles of the larynx are supplied by recurrent laryngeal nerve except cricothyroid, which gets its innervation from external laryngeal nerve.

(e) According to Semon's law, in case of progressive lesion of the recurrent laryngeal nerve, abductors are paralysed first while adductors are first to recover.

279. Tongue–I

(a) It is highly mobile muscular organ which is concerned with mastication, deglutition, taste, speech and oral cleansing.

(b) It consists of a root, a tip, two margins, dorsum and inferior surface.

(c) Its dorsum is divided into anterior two-thirds (oral part) and posterior one-third (pharyngeal part) by the V-shaped sulcus terminalis and foramen caecum.

(d) The papillae (vallate, fungiform and filiform) are confined to posterior one-third of its dorsum.

(e) Taste buds are widely spread over dorsum and sides of tongue, epiglottis and lingual surface of the soft palate.

280. Tongue–II

(a) Its extrinsic muscles converge to it from superior genial tubercle (genioglossus), styloid process (styloglossus), body and greater cornu of hyoid (hyoglossus), soft palate (palatoglossus) and lesser cornu of hyoid (chondroglossus).

(b) It is supplied by the branches of external carotid artery (lingual, facial and ascending pharyngeal).

(c) Deep lingual vein joins the sublingual vein to form vena comitans nervi hypoglossi, which unites with the dorsal lingual veins to form lingual vein.

(d) Lymphatics from its anterior, middle and posterior parts drain into submental, submandibular and jugulodigastric lymph nodes, respectively.

(e) In cases of paralysis of genioglossus, it deviates to the normal side during protrusion.

281. External acoustic meatus

(a) Ceruminous glands (secreting wax) and hair follicles (prone to infection) are largely confined to its cartilaginous part.

(b) Its blood supply comes from deep auricular branch of maxillary and auricular branches of superficial temporal arteries.

(c) The innervation of its anterosuperior wall is derived from auriculotemporal branch of mandibular nerve while the nerve supply for its posteroinferior wall comes from auricular branch of the vagus.

(d) To straighten the canal of the meatus, the auricle is pulled upwards, forwards.

(e) Its innervation by the vagus explains the occurrence of reflex coughing, sneezing and vomiting following the ear syringing.

282. Tympanic membrane

(a) It is derived from all the three embryonic layers (ecto-, endo- and mesoderm).

(b) Its concave lateral surface is directed downwards, laterally and backwards.

(c) It is divided into an upper smaller, pars flaccida and a lower larger, pars tensa by anterior and posterior malleolar folds.

(d) The arterial supply for its outer stratum is derived from deep auricular branch of maxillary artery while its inner mucosa is supplied by stylomastoid branch of occipital or posterior auricular artery.

(e) Its external surface is innervated by auricular branch of vagus and auriculotemporal nerve while internally it is supplied by tympanic branch of IX cranial nerve.

283. Middle ear–I

(a) In relation to the tympanic membrane, its cavity is divided into 3 parts, epitympanum (attic), mesotympanum and hypotympanum.

(b) It is narrowest (2 mm) opposite umbo of tympanic membrane and widest (6 mm) in its upper part.

(c) Its medial wall is marked by promontory, fenestra vestibuli (oval window), fenestra cochleae (round window) and the elevations produced by facial nerve and lateral semicircular canal.

(d) The lower part of its anterior wall has two openings (upper one for tensor tympani and lower one for Eustachian tube) and upper part of its anterior wall contains carotid canal.

(e) Its roof and floor are related to tegmen tympani and jugular fossa, respectively.

284. Middle ear–II

(a) Its three ossicles, from medial to lateral, are malleus, incus and stapes.

(b) Its mucosal folds constitute the anatomical barriers for spread of infection.

(c) It is innervated by tympanic plexus, which lies over the promontory and is contributed mainly by tympanic branch of IX cranial nerve.

(d) Its lateral wall is traversed by the chorda tympani.

(e) Tensor tympani is attached to the upper end of handle of malleus.

285. Mastoid antrum

(a) It communicates anteriorly with epitympanic recess through aditus to antrum and behind and below with the mastoid air cells.

(b) The suprameatal (Macewen's) triangle serves as a surgical landmark for the lateral wall of mastoid antrum, which is only 2 mm thick at birth but its thickness increases at the rate of 1 mm per year to attain the adult thickness of 12-15 mm.

(c) Its inflammation may involve the sigmoid sinus which lies in its posterior wall.

(d) Its anteroinferior relation is formed by the canal for facial nerve.

(e) Its roof is formed by tegmen tympani which separates it from posterior cranial fossa and occipital lobe.

286. Inner ear–I (osseous labyrinth)

(a) Its cavity is filled with perilymph and opens into middle ear through fenestrae vestibuli and cochleae which are closed by foot process of stapes and secondary tympanic membrane, respectively.

(b) Its cochlea consists of two and three quarter spiral turns of a tapering cylindrical canal.

(c) The base of modiolus, which is the axial bony stem for cochlea, lies at the promontory of middle ear.

(d) Its middle portion, the vestibule, contains the membranous saccule and utricle.

(e) The three semicircular canals, superior (anterior), posterior and lateral, lie in three different planes at right angle to one another.

287. Inner ear–II (membranous labyrinth)

(a) Its fluid, called endolymph, is separated from the perilymph of scala vestibuli and scala tympani by basilar and Reissner's membranes, respectively.

(b) Cochlear duct occupies the cochlea and is responsible for perception of hearing.

(c) Saccule and utricle maintain the static balance of body.

(d) The ducts of the semicircular canals take care of the kinetic balance.

(e) Spiral organ of Corti, located throughout the cochlear duct, consists of sound receptors and supporting cells covered by the membrana tectoria.

288. Eyeball–I (wall)

(a) The sclera is thickest (about 1 mm) posteriorly near the lamina cribrosa and is thinnest (about 0.4 mm) nearly 6 mm behind the corneoscleral junction.

(b) The cornea is convex anteriorly and this curvature is greater in younger age group than in elderly people.

(c) The choroid proper lies internal to the suprachoroid lamina and is composed of three laminae; internal vascular, intermediate capillary and external basal.

(d) Ciliary muscles and constrictor pupillae are innervated by the parasympathetic fibres while dilator pupillae are supplied by the sympathetic nerves.

(e) The retina is thickest (0.56 mm) near the optic disc and its thickness diminishes to 0.1 mm anterior to equator and it is thinnest at the fovea of macula.

289. Eyeball–II (refractive media)

(a) Interference with resorption of aqueous humour increases the intraocular pressure, a condition known as glaucoma.

(b) The lens is a transparent biconvex body with posterior convexity of greater radius than anterior one.

(c) In cataract, the lens gradually becomes opaque leading ultimately to blindness.

(d) The diameter of lens is 6.5 mm at birth and it gradually becomes 9 mm by the age of 15 years.

(e) Hyaloid canal, running from optic disc to the centre of posterior surface of the lens, contains hyaloid artery in foetal life which disappears about 6 weeks before birth.

ABDOMEN AND PELVIS

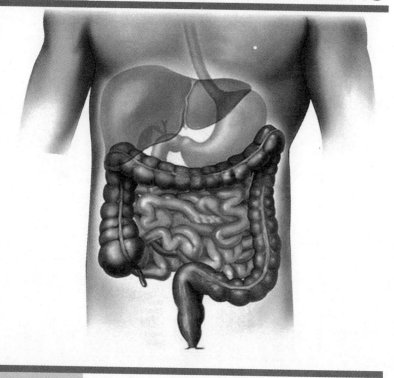

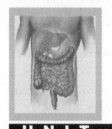

ABDOMEN AND PELVIS

6

Find out incorrect statement in each set.

290. Introduction to abdomen and pelvis–I

(a) It is part of trunk below the diaphragm.

(b) It is divisible into abdomen proper and pelvis by the plane of pelvic inlet.

(c) False pelvis corresponds with the lower part of abdomen proper.

(d) Midinguinal point is the midpoint of the line between anterior superior iliac spine and pubic symphysis.

(e) Midpoint of inguinal ligament is a point on the inguinal ligament between anterior superior iliac spine and pubic tubercle.

291. Introduction to abdomen and pelvis–II

(a) Transpyloric (Addison's) plane passes through the tips of 9th costal cartilages and corresponds with upper border of 1st lumbar vertebra.

(b) Subcostal plane passes through intervertebral disc between lumbar vertebrae 2 and 3.

(c) Transumbilical or supracristal planes lie at the level of intervertebral disc between lumbar vertebrae 3 and 4.

(d) Transtubercular plane runs through intervertebral disc between lumbar vertebrae 4 and 5.

(e) Lateral (right and left) vertical plane passes through midpoint of clavicle above and midinguinal point below.

292. Introduction to abdomen and pelvis–III

(a) The planes dividing the abdomen into 9 regions, are two vertical (right and left) and two horizontal (transpyloric and transtubercular).

(b) Out of 9 abdominal regions, 3 are unpaired (epigastric, umbilical and hypogastric) and 3 paired (hypochondriac, lumbar and inguinal).

(c) Division of abdomen into 4 quadrants is based on median and supracristal planes.

(d) Viscera lying in four quadrants are liver and gallbladder in the upper left, stomach and spleen in the upper right, caecum and appendix in the lower right while descending and sigmoid colon in lower left region.

(e) According to RW Mill's classification, bodily habitus can be divided into 4 groups—hypersthenic (5%), sthenic (48%), hyposthenic (35%) and asthenic (12%).

293. Superficial structures of anterior abdominal wall–I

(a) Incisions along the horizontally disposed Langer's lines in the skin, heal with hair-line scar.

(b) Anterior cutaneous branches of lower 5 and lateral cutaneous branches of lower 2 intercostal nerves mainly supply the skin.

(c) Subcostal (T_{12}) and iliohypogastric (L_1) nerves, being purely muscular, do not supply the skin.

(d) Anterior and lateral cutaneous arteries emerge from epigastric (superior and inferior) and lumbar arteries, respectively.

(e) Circumflex iliac (superficial and deep), superficial epigastric and external pudendal (superficial and deep) arteries are additional cutaneous twigs for lower abdomen and external genitalia.

294. Superficial structures of anterior abdominal wall–II

(a) Cutaneous veins diverge from umbilicus to great saphenous and lateral thoracic veins.

(b) Caput medusae results form the obstruction of paraumbilical veins.

(c) A vertical dilated venous channel makes its appearance on each side of the front of trunk in case of vena caval obstruction.

(d) Superficial lymphatics above and below the umbilicus drain into axillary and superficial inguinal lymph nodes, respectively.

(e) Malignancy of umbilicus may lead to enlargement of axillary and superficial inguinal lymph nodes of both the sides simultaneously.

295. Superficial structures of anterior abdominal wall–III (superficial fascia)

(a) Above the umbilicus, it is single layer of fatty connective tissue.

(b) Below the umbilicus, it is divisible into a superficial membranous layer (of Scarpa) and deep fatty layer (of Camper).

(c) The fascia of Camper and Scarpa correspond with the panniculus adiposus and carnosus respectively in lower animals.

(d) Colles' fascia is the continuation of fascia of Scarpa into the perineum.

(e) Extravasated urine after urethral rupture does not extend into the thigh due to attachment of facia of Scarpa with the fascia lata along Holden's line.

296. Anterolateral abdominal muscles–I (external oblique)

(a) It originates from lower 6 ribs.

(b) It gets inserted by its muscle to anterior half of iliac crest and by its aponeurosis to anterior superior iliac spine, pubic tubercle, rectus sheath and linea alba.

(c) It is innervated by lower intercostals (T_7-T_{11}) and subcostal nerves.

(d) It superior, posterior and inferior margins are free, the latter is known as inguinal (Poupart's) ligament.

(e) Superficial inguinal ring is a triangular gap in its aponeurosis.

297. Anterolateral abdominal muscles–II (internal oblique)

(a) It originates from lateral two-thirds of inguinal ligament, anterior two-thirds of ventral segment of iliac crest and thoracolumbar fascia.

(b) It gets inserted to pubic crest (via conjoint tendon), rectus sheath and linea alba.

(c) It is innervated by lower intercostals (T_7-T_{11}), subcostal (T_{12}) and iliohypogastric (L_1) nerves.

(d) The plane between this muscle and external oblique forms neurovascular plane.

(e) It is pierced by iliohypogastric nerve 2 cm medial to anterior superior iliac spine.

298. Anterolateral abdominal muscles–III (transversus abdominis)

(a) It originates from lateral one-third of inguinal ligament, anterior two-thirds of ventral segment of iliac crest, thoracolumbar fascia and lower 6 costal cartilages.

(b) It gets inserted to pubic crest (via conjoint tendon) and contributes to rectus sheath and linea al–11), subcostal (T_{12}) and iliohypogastric (L_1) nerves.

· (c) Its costal fibres interdigitate with those of latissimus dorsi.

(d) Transversalis fascia is a thin connective tissue layer between this muscle and extraperitoneal fat.

299. Anterolateral abdominal muscle–IV (rectus abdominis)

(a) It originates by its medial and lateral tendons from the pubic symphysis and pubic crest, respectively.

(b) It is inserted over the 3rd, 4th and 5th costal cartilages.

(c) It is innervated by lower intercostals (T_7–T_{11}) and subcostal nerves.

(d) Pyramidalis (from pubic crest to linea alba) covering its lower part, is supplied by subcostal nerve.

(e) It is an important flexor of vertebral column.

300. Rectus sheath

(a) It is a fibrous compartment with complete posterior wall and incomplete anterior wall.

(b) It increases the efficiency of rectus abdominis by keeping it in position.

(c) It encloses muscles (rectus abdominis and pyramidalis), vessels (superior and inferior epigastric) and nerves (lower five intercostals and subcostal).

(d) Aponeuroses of flat muscles contributing to it are bilaminar making its walls trilaminar.

(e) Aponeurotic layer in the rectus sheath of one side continues with some other layer of the opposite side giving rise to the concept of bilateral digastric muscles.

301. Inguinal canal–I

(a) It is located above the medial part of inguinal ligament and lacunar ligament, which therefore form its floor.

(b) It measures about 4 cm.

(c) Its anterior wall is formed by aponeurosis of external oblique throughout and internal oblique in its lateral part only.

(d) Its posterior wall is formed by fascia transversalis throughout and conjoint tendon and reflected inguinal ligament in its medial part only.

(e) Its roof is formed by arched fibres of internal oblique.

302. Inguinal canal–II

(a) It extends from deep inguinal ring (in fascia transversalis) to superficial inguinal ring (in aponeurosis of internal oblique).

(b) It is occupied by spermatic cord in male and round ligament of uterus in female.

(c) Superficial and deep inguinal rings are strengthened by falx inguinalis and internal oblique, respectively.

(d) Contraction of internal oblique produces traction on deep inguinal ring and thus responsible for valvular safety mechanism.

(e) Direct inguinal hernia takes place through Hesselbach's triangle.

303. Spermatic cord

(a) It is located partly in the abdominal cavity and partly in the inguinal canal.

(b) Its 3 arteries are testicular artery, artery of vas deferens and cremasteric artery.

(c) The veins accompanying the testicular artery in the scrotum form pampiniform plexus.

(d) Its three nervous components are sympathetic fibres, genital branch of genitofemoral nerve and ilioinguinal nerve.

(e) Vasectomy is the commonest surgical procedure to produce male sterility.

304. Scrotum

(a) Dortos muscle replaces subcutaneous fat in its wall.

(b) All its layers except skin (dortos and fasciae-external spermatic, cremasteric and internal spermatic) contribute to the septum.

(c) Temperature of testis is maintained by counter current heat exchange between venous (pampiniform plexus) and arterial (testicular artery) blood.

(d) Anterior one-third of its skin is supplied by scrotal nerve (S_3) while posterior two-thirds is innervated by ilioinguinal nerve (L_1).

(e) Hydrocele results from the collection of excess fluid in the tunica vaginalis.

305. Testis

(a) Gubernaculum testis and differential growth of body are two important factors helping the descent of testis.

(b) Its length, width and thickness is approximately 5, 3 and 2.5 cm, respectively.

(c) It weighs about 25 g.

(d) It has two surfaces (medial and lateral), two margins (anterior and posterior) and two poles (superior and inferior).

(e) Testicular pain is referred to umbilicus due to same segmental innervation (T_{10}).

306. Peritoneum–I

(a) Fold of peritoneum connecting the mobile viscera with abdominal wall is called mesentery.

(b) Peritoneal fold connecting stomach with the adjacent viscus is called ligament.

(c) The greater and lesser sacs communicate with each other through epiploic foramen (foramen of Winslow).

(d) Both falciform ligament and lesser omentum are derived from ventral mesogastrium.

(e) Hepatorenal pouch of Morison is the most dependant part of peritoneal cavity in the abdomen proper during supine posture.

307. Peritoneum–II

(a) Lubrication, storage of fat, support of viscera and resisting the infection, are some of its important functions.

(b) Greater omentum is also called abdominal police man due to its property of covering the viscera.

(c) Pelvic peritoneum is innervated by obturator nerve.

(d) Pain of parietal peritoneum is severe and precisely localized while that of visceral one is dull and poorly localized.

(e) Collection of fluid in the peritoneal cavity is called ascites.

308. Peritoneum–III (lesser sac)

(a) It is located behind the stomach and greater omentum.

(b) Its superior, inferior and left borders extend to diaphragm, greater omentum and spleen, respectively.

(c) Its right border has foramen of Winslow.

(d) Free margin of lesser omentum (with portal vein, bile duct and hepatic artery) forms the anterior border of foramen of Winslow.

(e) It may be the site for internal abdominal hernia.

309. Stomach–I

(a) It is the most dilated part of the gut between oesophagus and duodenum.

(b) It occupies left hypochondriac, epigastric and umbilical regions.

(c) Its distal opening, called as pyloric orifice, is marked by well-developed anatomical sphincter.

(d) Its proximal opening called as cardiac orifice, is said to have physiological sphincter due to its sphincteric behaviour in the absence of well-developed circular fibres.

(e) Its lesser and greater curvatures are directed towards left and right side, respectively.

310. Stomach–II

(a) Magenblaze is the gas in its fundus.

(b) Magenstrasse or gastric canal is a narrow temporary tunnel along the lesser curvature produced by the contraction of its oblique fibres.

(c) Its capacities at birth, puberty and adult are 1, 1.5 and 2 litres, respectively.

(d) Greater omentum can be further divided into gastrophrenic, gastrosplenic and gastrocolic ligaments.

(e) Transverse colon and mesocolon, pancreas, kidney (left), suprarenal gland (left), diaphragm, spleen and splenic artery form stomach bed.

311. Stomach–III

(a) Temporary storage, mixing, partial digestion and absorption are its important functions.

(b) It produces intrinsic factor, which combines with extrinsic factor (B_{12}) to form a hemopoietic factor.

(c) There are many gastric (right, left, short and posterior) and two gastroepiploic (right and left) arteries for its supply.

(d) Gastroepiploic arteries adjoin its greater curvature.

(e) Its veins accompany the arteries and drain, directly or indirectly into the portal vein.

312. Stomach–IV

(a) All its lymphatics ultimately drain into coeliac lymph nodes.

(b) It receives parasympathetic fibres from anterior and posterior vagal trunks which are derived mainly from right and left vagi, respectively.

(c) Parasympathetic fibres are motor to glands and muscles while inhibitory to pylorus.

(d) Sympathetic fibres (T_6–T_9), derived from greater and lesser splanchnic nerves, reach the stomach via coeliac plexus along its arteries.

(e) Sympathetic fibres are motor to vessels and pylorus.

313. Spleen–I

(a) It extends from side of vertebral column to midaxillary line along 9th to 11th ribs on the left side.

(b) It develops in the left leaf of dorsal mesogastrium during 7th week of intrauterine life.

(c) It has superior, inferior and notched anterior borders.

(d) Its weight is about 150 g.

(e) Its visceral surface has gastric, renal, colic and pancreatic impressions.

314. Spleen–II

(a) Its important functions are phagocytosis, immune response, cytopoiesis and erythrocyte storage.

(b) It is drained by pancreaticosplenic lymph nodes located in its hilum.

(c) Its nerves, derived from coeliac plexus, are vasomotor in nature.

(d) Majority (85%) shows three segments (superior, intermediate and inferior) while minority (16%) represents only two segments (superior and inferior) in it.

(e) Referred pain in the left shoulder due to irritation of phrenic nerve by the discharge from ruptured spleen is called Kehr's sign.

315. Small intestine–I

(a) It extends from gastroduodenal junction to ileocaecal junction.

(b) First 25 cm of small intestine is duodenum.

(c) Duodenum is divisible into superior (5 cm), descending (7.5 cm), horizontal (10 cm) and ascending (2.5) parts.

(d) Excluding the duodenum, rest of the small intestine (6 m) is divisible into proximal 2/5th (jejunum) and distal 3/5th (ileum).

(e) Gastroduodenal junction is marked by the attachment of ligament of Treitz.

316. Small intestine–II

(a) Only duodenum beyond its 1st 2.5 cm, is retroperitoneal, while rest of the small intestine is mobile.

(b) The attached margin (root) of the mesentery (holding jejunum and ileum) extends from the left side of 1st lumbar vertebra to right sacroiliac joint.

(c) Length of the root of mesentery is about 15 cm.

(d) The root of mesentery crosses duodenum, aorta, inferior vena cava, right ureter and right psoas (DAVUP).

(e) Average width of the mesentery is 20 cm.

317. Small intestine–III

(a) 1st and 2nd parts of duodenum lie on the right side of 1st two lumbar vertebrae, the 3rd part crosses the 2nd lumbar vertebra, while 4th part is related to the left side of 1st lumbar vertebra.

(b) The concavity of duodenum is occupied by the head of pancreas.

(c) The descending part of duodenum is related anteriorly to gall-bladder, liver, intestinal coils, transverse colon and transverse mesocolon (GLITT).

(d) Posteromedial wall of the interior of 2nd part of duodenum has got major and minor duodenal papillae.

(e) The front of the 3rd part of duodenum is related to the mesentery (root), superior mesenteric vessels and coils of jejunum (MSC).

318. Small intestine–IV

(a) Jejunum can be differentiated from ileum on the basis of thick mucosa, wide lumen, few arterial arcades and long vasa recta.

(b) Ileal (Meckel's) diverticulum is persistence of intra-abdominal part of allantoic diverticulum.

(c) Ileal diverticulum is found in 3% individuals, about 100 cm proximal to ileocaecal junction and is 5 cm in length (THREE HUNDRED FIVE).

(d) Meckelian diverticulitis resembles appendicitis in its presentation.

(e) Littre's hernia is inguinal hernia with Meckel's diverticulum as its content.

319. Small intestine–V

(a) Coeliac trunk supplies up to the middle of 2nd part of duodenum, while superior mesenteric artery supplies rest of the small intestine.

(b) All the veins draining the small intestine join portal vein directly or indirectly via superior mesenteric vein.

   (c) Prepyloric vein, a surgical guide to pylorus, drains into superior mesenteric vein.

   (d) Upper duodenum is drained by celiac lymph nodes while rest of the small intestine is drained by superior mesenteric lymph nodes.

   (e) Lymphatics draining the jejunum and ileum are interrupted by mesenteric lymph nodes (mural, intermediate and juxta-arterial).

320. Small intestine–VI

   (a) It receives both sympathetic (T_9–T_{10}) and parasympathetic fibres (Vagus).

   (b) Autonomic fibres for upper duodenum are derived from celiac plexus while those for the rest of small intestine come from superior mesenteric plexus.

   (c) Duodenal ulcer commonly involves its posterior wall.

   (d) Perforation of duodenal ulcer in its posterior wall may lead to profuse bleeding due to erosion of gastroduodenal artery.

   (e) A tumour or cyst of the mesentery is more mobile across its attachment.

321. Pancreas–I

   (a) Its length is about 20–25 cm.

   (b) It is divisible into head (with uncinate process), neck (2 cm), body and tail.

   (c) Superior mesenteric vessels lie in front of uncinate process.

   (d) Its neck is crossed in front by gastroduodenal artery and behind by superior mesenteric and portal veins.

   (e) Its body is related posteriorly with diaphragm (left crus), aorta, renal vessels (left), kidney (left), superior mesenteric artery, suprarenal gland (left) and splenic vein (DARK SSS).

322. Pancreas–II

   (a) Its tail enters the splenorenal ligament to reach the spleen.

(b) Main pancreatic and common bile ducts unite to form ampulla of Vater (with sphincter of Oddi) which opens at the summit of major duodenal papilla.

(c) Its head is supplied by pancreaticoduodenal arteries (superior and inferior) while rest is supplied by splenic artery.

(d) Parasympathetic fibres (right vagus) supply its parenchyma only while sympathetic fibres (T_7–T_9) are also vasomotor in addition to its parenchymal supply.

(e) Cancer of head leads to diabetes mellitus.

323. Large intestine–I

(a) Its total length is about 155 cm.

(b) The 1st part of the colon (ascending colon) and last part of large intestine (rectum and anal canal) are equal in lengths, i.e. 15 cm each.

(c) The part of the colon having mesenteries (transverse and sigmoid) equal in their lengths, i.e. 45 cm each.

(d) The length of descending colon is the mean of those of ascending colon and transverse colon, i.e. 30 cm.

(e) The width of caecum (6 cm) is less than its height (7.5 cm).

324. Large intestine–II

(a) Large lumen, taeniae coli, sacculations and appendices epiploicae differentiate caecum and colon from rest of the alimentary canal.

(b) Type II (quadrate) caecum is observed in majority of individuals.

(c) Retrocaecal (12 o'clock) and pelvic (4 o'clock) positions of vermiform appendix are commonly observed, i.e. in 65% and 31% individuals, respectively.

(d) Less common positions of appendix are 1 o'clock (postileal), 2 o'clock (preileal), 3 o'clock (promontoric), 6 o'clock (subcaecal) and 11 o'clock (paracaecal).

(e) All three taeneae coli converge at the base of appendix, an information of surgical importance.

325. Large intestine–III

(a) Mesoappendix is derived from the right leaf of the mesentery.

(b) 48% individuals show either ascending mesocolon or descending mesocolon or both.

(c) Sigmoid mesocolon is inverted 'V' (^) shaped, the limbs of which measure 5 cm each.

(d) Caecum rests over two muscles (psoas, iliacus), two nerves (lateral cutaneous nerve of thigh and femoral) and two vessels (external iliac and gonadal).

(e) Ascending colon lies over four muscles (psoas, iliacus, quadratus lumborum and transversus abdominis), two nerves (ilioinguinal and iliohypogastric) and right kidney.

326. Large intestine–IV

(a) Caecum and appendix are supplied by caecal (anterior and posterior) and appendicular arteries from inferior branch of ileocolic twig of superior mesenteric artery.

(b) Marginal artery of Drummond is formed by the colic branches of the superior and inferior mesenteric arteries.

(c) The large intestine proximal to the junction of right two-thirds with the left one-third of transverse colon (midgut) is drained by superior mesenteric vein while rest (hindgut) by inferior mesenteric vein.

(d) Lymphatics of midgut and hindgut portions of colon drain into inferior and superior mesenteric lymph nodes, respectively.

(e) Lymphatics from colon are interrupted by colic (epicolic, paracolic, intermediate colic and preterminal colic) lymph nodes.

327. Large intestine–V

(a) Its midgut portion is supplied by superior mesenteric plexus while its hindgut part is innervated by inferior mesenteric plexus.

(b) Its sympathetic fibres are derived from thoracic splanchnic nerves (T_{10}–T_{11}) where as parasympathetic fibres for its midgut portion come from vagus while those for hindgut part emerge from hypogastric plexus (S_2–S_4).

(c) Pain from appendix is referred to umbilicus due to identical segmental innervation (T_{10}).

(d) Diverticulosis is evagination of the whole thickness of the intestinal wall.

(e) In cases of large bowel obstruction, the caecum is full of faeces.

328. Portal vein–I

(a) Its length is approximately 15 cm.

(b) It is formed by the union of superior mesenteric and splenic veins between the neck of pancreas and inferior vena cava.

(c) It terminates into right and left branches at porta hepatis.

(d) It ascends first behind the first part of duodenum and then in the free margin of lesser omentum.

(e) It drains the alimentary canal (from lower end of oesophagus to anal canal), pancreas, spleen and gallbladder.

329. Portal vein–II

(a) In addition to two veins at its commencement, it receives gastric (right and left), paraumbilical and cystic veins.

(b) Its obstruction leads to hepatomegaly, ascites and varicose veins at the sites of portosystemic anastomoses.

(c) Varicose veins at the lower one-third of oesophagus are called oesophageal varices.

(d) Dilated and tortuous (varicose) veins in the anal canal are termed as haemorrhoids.

(e) Portal obstruction makes the radiating veins around the umbilicus dilated and tortuous, a condition called caput medusae.

330. Liver–I

(a) It is the largest gland in the body.

(b) Its weight is approximately 1.5 kg.

(c) It is located mainly in the left hypochondriac and epigastric regions of abdomen.

(d) It has five surfaces—posterior, anterior, right, superior and inferior (PARSI).

(e) Its only well-defined border is inferior which intervenes between anterior and inferior surfaces.

331. Liver–II

(a) Falciform ligament connects its anterosuperior surface with the anterior abdominal wall and diaphragm.

(b) The peritoneal folds attached to its posterior surface are lesser omentum, coronary ligament and triangular (right and left) ligaments.

(c) Diaphragm separates it from pleural and pericardial cavities.

(d) Three concavities on its posterior aspect are related to (from right to left) oesophagus, vertebral column and inferior vena cava.

(e) Its visceral surface is related to kidney (right), gallbladder, duodenum, stomach and colic flexure (right).

332. Liver–III

(a) Attachment of falciform ligament forms the basis for its anatomical right and left lobes.

(b) Plane of inferior vena cava and gallbladder splits it into physiological right and left lobes.

(c) Its right lobe (physiological) is further divided into medial, intermediate and lateral segments.

(d) Its left lobe (physiological) is further divided into medial part (3 regions—anterior, central and posterior) and lateral part (2 segments—anterior and posterior).

(e) Gupta divided the liver into 5 segments – right, middle, left, caudate and paracaval.

333. Liver–IV

(a) It receives 80% blood from hepatic artery while 20% blood from portal vein.

(b) Hepatic veins (2–3) drain their blood into inferior vena cava.

(c) Both its superficial and deep lymphatics drain mainly into coeliac and hepatic lymph nodes.

(d) Its parasympathetic fibres are derived from both the vagal trunks while sympathetic fibres (T_7–T_9) reach it via greater splanchnic nerves and coeliac plexus.

(e) Cancer and hydatid cyst may lead to massive hepatomegaly. -

334. Extrahepatic biliary apparatus–I

(a) The capacity of gallbladder is approximately 40 ml.

(b) Gallbladder is divisible into fundus, body, infundibulum (with Hartmann's pouch) and neck.

(c) Cystic artery most commonly arises from left hepatic artery.

(d) The function of gallbladder is to store and concentrate the bile.

(e) Referred right shoulder pain in gallbladder pathology is due to its supply by the phrenic nerve via its communication with coeliac plexus which provides autonomic fibres to it.

335. Extrahepatic biliary apparatus–II

(a) Cystic duct about 3.5 cm in length, connects the neck of gall-bladder with the common hepatic duct.

(b) Common bile duct is about 15 cm in length.

(c) Common bile duct is divisible into three parts—supraduodenal, retroduodenal and infraduodenal.

(d) Upper part of common bile duct is supplied by cystic artery while its lower part is supplied by posterior superior pancreaticoduodenal artery.

(e) Sphincter of Boyden is located at the lower end of common bile duct just proximal to its union with the pancreatic duct.

336. Diaphragm–I

(a) It is a musculotendinous partition between thorax and abdomen.

(b) It originates from xiphoid, costal margin, lumbar vertebrae (upper three) and arcuate ligaments (median, medial and lateral).

(c) Its fibres converge towards the central tendon which is trefoil and comprised of central part and three leaves (right, left and anterior).

(d) It is supplied by inferior phrenic arteries from below and musculophrenic and pericardiacophrenic arteries from above.

(e) It helps in peristaltic movements, foetal movements and yawning.

337. Diaphragm–II

(a) Aortic aperture (level–T_{12}) provides passage to vena azygos, aorta, lymphatics and thoracic duct (VALT).

(b) Structures passing through oesophageal aperture (level–T_{10}) are—vagal trunks (anterior and posterior), oesophagus, oesophageal vessels and lymphatics (VOOL).

(c) Vena caval aperture (level–T_8) allows passage of lymphatics, inferior vena cava and phrenic (right) nerve (VP).

(d) Its motor supply is derived from lower intercostal (T_7–T_{11}) nerves while sensory fibres come from phrenic nerves.

(e) Sliding is the commonest type (85%) of hiatus hernia whereas rolling type or mixed picture is observed in 10% and 5% cases, respectively.

338. Posterior wall of abdomen–I (quadratus lumborum)

(a) It originates from posterior one-third of the inner lip of the ventral segment of iliac crest as well as lower lumbar transverse processes.

(b) It is inserted on the medial half of the lower part of the anterior surface of 12th rib as well as upper lumbar transverse processes.

(c) It is supplied by the ventral rami of upper 4 lumbar nerves.

(d) It helps in lateral flexion of spine as well as respiration.

(e) It is covered by the anterior and posterior layers of thoracolumbar fascia.

339. Posterior wall of abdomen–II (iliopsoas)

(a) Psoas major extends from bodies and transverse processes of lumbar vertebrae to lesser trochanter of femur.

(b) Iliacus extends from iliac fossa to lesser trochanter of femur.

(c) Iliopsoas is innervated by femoral nerve.

(d) Anteromedial margin of psoas major is in contact with sympathetic trunk.

(e) Iliopsoas causes flexion and medial rotation of thigh while psoas major additionally produces lateral flexion of spine.

340. Posterior wall of abdomen–III (nerves)

(a) It is comprised of subcostal nerve (T_{12}), lumbar plexus (L_1–L_4), sympathetic chain and autonomic plexuses.

(b) Subcostal nerve enters the abdomen by passing deep to lateral arcuate ligament.

(c) Ilioinguinal (L_1), anterior branch of iliohypogastric (L_1), genitofemoral (L_1, L_2) and obturator (L_2–L_4) nerves arise from the ventral divisions of lumbar plexus.

(d) Dorsal divisions of lumbar plexus provide lateral branch of iliohypogastric (L_1), lateral cutaneous nerve of thigh (L_2, L_3) and femoral nerve (L_2–L_4).

(e) Obturator nerve descends on the anterior aspect of psoas major.

341. Posterior wall of abdomen–IV (autonomic nerves)

(a) There are 5 lumbar and 5 sacral sympathetic ganglia on each side but only one ganglion impar in front of coccyx.

(b) White rami communicantes appear from upper two lumbar ganglia while grey rami communicantes emerge from all the ganglia.

    (c) Lumbar splanchnic nerves join hypogastric plexus.

    (d) Most of the abdominal autonomic plexuses are named after aorta (abdominal aortic plexus) or its branches (coeliac, phrenic, left gastric, splenic, hepatic, renal, superior and inferior mesenteric plexuses).

    (e) Lumbar sympathectomy (removal of 2nd to 4th sympathetic ganglia), is done in cases of Buerger's disease.

342. Posterior wall of abdomen–V (abdominal aorta)

    (a) It extends from the aortic hiatus in the diaphragm (level T_{12}) to the level of the body of 4th lumbar vertebra.

    (b) It provides three ventral unpaired arteries—coeliac and superior and inferior mesenteric.

    (c) Its lateral paired branches are—inferior phrenic, superior suprarenal, renal and gonadal arteries.

    (d) Branches appearing from its dorsal aspect are 4 pairs of lumbar and single median sacral arteries.

    (e) It terminates, at the level of 4th lumbar vertebral body, into two common iliac arteries.

343. Posterior wall of abdomen–VI (inferior vena cava and lymphatic system)

    (a) Inferior vena cava extends from 5th lumbar vertebral body to vena caval orifice in the diaphragm (level–T_8).

    (b) Paired tributaries of inferior vena cava are common iliac, lumbar, gonadal and renal veins.

    (c) Inferior vena cava receives all the hepatic veins (usually 3) but inferior phrenic and suprarenal veins from right side only.

    (d) Abdominal lymph nodes are usually named after the vessels, e.g. aortic: (pre, lateral, retro) and iliac: (common, external, internal).

    (e) Cisterna chyli, a lymphatic sac lying over upper two lumbar vertebrae, receives one intestinal trunk (draining the digestive system) and two lumbar trunks (draining the walls and urogenital system).

344. Suprarenal gland–I

(a) It weighs about 5 g.

(b) It is enclosed in perinephric fat and renal fascia.

(c) Right suprarenal is crescentic in shape while left one is pyramidal.

(d) Posterior relations are same (diaphragm and corresponding kidney) for both the glands whereas anterior relations are inferior vena cava and liver for right gland and stomach and pancreas for left one.

(e) Three suprarenal arteries, i.e. superior, middle and inferior, are derived from inferior phrenic, aorta and renal arteries, respectively.

345. Suprarenal gland–II

(a) Single vein appears from the hilum of each gland and drains on the right side into renal vein while on left side into inferior vena cava.

(b) Its lymphatics enter into lateral aortic lymph nodes.

(c) Preganglionic sympathetic fibres (T_{10}–L_1) supply the gland via coeliac plexus.

(d) Reduction in its cortical secretions leads to Addison's disease while increase in the same results into Cushing's syndrome.

(e) Tumour from its medulla (pheochromocytoma) is responsible for secondary hypertension.

346. Kidney–I

(a) Its weight is approximately 140 g.

(b) Its length, width and thickness are 11, 6 and 3 cm, respectively.

(c) Its hilum is located 5 cm from midline in transpyloric plane.

(d) Renal fascia intervenes between its capsule and perinephric fat.

(e) Kidney rests over 4 muscles (quadratus lumborum, diaphragm, psoas, transversus abdominis), 3 nerves (subcostal, iliohypogastric, ilioinguinal), 2 ribs (11th and 12th) and two vessel (subcostal).

347. Kidney–II

(a) Renal artery divides into anterior and posterior divisions and the former further spits into 4 branches to supply the kidney.

(b) Graves' vascular segments of kidney are—apical, superior, middle, inferior and posterior.

(c) Brodel's bloodless line is located near the lateral border of kidney on its posterior surface.

(d) Sympathetic fibres (T_{12}–L_1) supplying the kidney are vasomotor in nature.

(e) In case of horseshoe kidney, the pelvis and ureter descend behind this organ.

348. Ureter–I

(a) It measures about 30 cm in length of which upper half is abdominal and lower half is pelvic.

(b) It descends over the psoas major along the margins of the lower 4 lumbar vertebral bodies.

(c) Both the ureters are crossed by corresponding gonadal and colic vessels.

(d) The duodenum and "the mesentery" are related to front of the right ureter only while sigmoid colon and mesocolon lie exclusively on the anterior aspect of left ureter.

(e) It can be marked on the surface of anterior abdominal wall by joining the hilum of kidney (on transpyloric plane, 5 cm from midline) with pubic tubercle.

349. Ureter–II

(a) It shows three constrictions—1st at commencement (at the tip of 2nd lumbar transverse process), 2nd in its middle (at pelvic brim) and 3rd at its lower end (little medial to ischial spine).

(b) Its abdominal part receives arterial supply from renal, abdominal, gonadal and common iliac arteries.

(c) Its pelvic part is supplied by middle rectal and median sacral arteries.

(d) It is drained, from above downwards by lateral aortic, common iliac, external iliac and internal iliac lymph nodes.

(e) Its innervation by sympathetic fibres from T_{10}–L_1 segments of spinal cord explains the referred pain in cases of renal colic to testis (T_{10}) or medial thigh (L_1).

350. Bony pelvis–I

(a) It is divided into true (lesser) pelvis and false (greater) pelvis by the pelvic diaphragm.

(b) The cavity of true pelvis is bounded by pubic symphysis and pubis anteriorly, sacrum posteriorly and pelvic surfaces of ilium and ischium laterally.

(c) The inlet of true pelvis is bounded anteriorly by superior margin of pubic symphysis, posteriorly by sacral promontory and on each side by pelvic brim.

(d) The pelvic brim is comprised of ala of sacrum and linea terminalis, the latter being contributed by arcuate line, pecten pubis and pubic crest.

(e) Inlet of true pelvis and pelvic brim are synonyms for obstetricians.

351. Bony pelvis–II

(a) Its outlet is formed anteriorly by lower border of pubic symphysis, posteriorly by tip of coccyx and on each side by ischiopubic ramus, ischial tuberosity and sacrotuberous ligament.

(b) Female pelvis can be divided into 4 types—gynecoid (22%), android (32%), anthropoid (42%) and platypelloid (2%).

(c) Inclinations of inlet and outlet are approximately 55° and 15°, respectively.

(d) All the diameters (anteroposterior, transverse and oblique) of the cavity and only oblique diameters of inlet and outlet, are same, i.e. about 12 cm.

(e) The anteroposterior diameters of inlet and outlet are 11 and 13 cm respectively while transverse diameters of the same are 13 and 11 cm, respectively.

352. Bony pelvis–III

(a) The inlet of true pelvis is divided into anterior and posterior segments by widest transverse diameter.

(b) The angle of the pubic arch in gynecoid pelvis is >90° (Norman type) while that of the android pelvis is <90° (Gothic type).

(c) Plane of greatest pelvic dimension passes from the middle of pubic symphysis to the junction of 2nd and 3rd sacral vertebrae.

(d) Plane of least pelvic dimension lies at the level of tip of sacrum, ischial spines and lower part of pubic symphysis.

(e) True conjugate and diagonal conjugate extend from sacral promontory to inferior and superior margins of pubic symphysis, respectively.

353. Pelvic wall–I (piriformis)

(a) Its three digitations originate from the pelvic surfaces of middle three pieces of sacrum.

(b) It passes through lesser sciatic foramen to enter the gluteal region.

(c) It gets inserted over the superior border of greater trochanter of femur.

(d) It is innervated by branches from L_5, S_1–S_2.

(e) It produces lateral rotation in extended thigh and abduction in flexed thigh.

354. Pelvic wall–II (obturator internus)

(a) It arises from the internal surface of obturator membrane and adjacent bones.

(b) It enters the gluteal region by passing through lesser sciatic foramen where it is accompanied by superior and inferior gemelli.

(c) Its tendon gets inserted into the trochanteric fossa.

(d) The nerve supplying it is named as nerve to obturator internus (L_5, S_1).

(e) This muscle along with the gemelli rotates laterally the extended thigh but abducts the flexed thigh.

355. Pelvic floor–I (pelvic diaphragm)

(a) It is formed by coccygeus (also called ischiococcygeus) and levator ani (comprised of iliococcygeus and pubococcygeus).

(b) Coccygeus is a triangular musculotendinous sheet extending from the apex of ischial spine to the side of coccyx and 5th sacral segment.

(c) Sacrospinous ligament is considered to be degenerated part of the coccygeus.

(d) Coccygeus is innervated by spinal nerves S_4, S_5.

(e) Coccygeus is often absent and sacrospinous ligament well developed in tailed mammals.

356. Pelvic diaphragm–II (levator ani)

(a) It originates from the body of pubis, tendinous arch over obturator fascia and ischial spine.

(b) Fibres from the anterior half of its origin form pubococcygeus and lie at a higher plane while those from the posterior half of its origin form iliococcygeus and lie at a lower plane.

(c) Pubococcygeus has three components—anterior fibres get attached to perineal body (puboprostaticus in male and pubovaginalis in female), intermediate fibres form puborectalis sling while the posterior fibres (pubococcygeus proper) form anococcygeal raphe.

(d) It is innervated from above by perineal branch of S_4 while from below by inferior rectal and perineal nerves.

(e) In tailed mammals, both of its components are attached to sacrum only.

357. Pelvic fascia

(a) According to location, it can be divided into 3 parts—parietal, visceral and fascia between the pelvic floor and peritoneum.

(b) Parietal pelvic fascia either lines the pelvic wall (obturator and piriform fasciae) or floor (superior fascia of pelvic diaphragm).

(c) Visceral pelvic fascia is well defined thick membrane over the distensible viscera but very thin over non-distensible viscera.

(d) At places it forms condensation around vessels and nerves (e.g. Mackenrodt's ligament, lateral ligament of bladder and fascia of Waldeyer).

(e) At places it is condensed to support the viscera (puboprostatic ligament, round ligament of uterus and uterosacral ligament).

358. Pelvic peritoneum–I

(a) It can be divided into parietal and visceral layers according to its relations.

(b) Its parietal layer is innervated by a branch from sacral plexus.

(c) After covering the sides and front of upper rectum, it is reflected over upper part of the back of urinary bladder in male, forming rectovesical pouch.

(d) Fascia of Denonvillier connects the rectovesical fold with the pelvic floor.

(e) It covers mainly the superior surface of urinary bladder.

359. Pelvic peritoneum–II

(a) It is reflected from the superior surface of urinary bladder to the back of lower part of anterior abdominal wall leaving an extraperitoneal space (cave of Retzius) behind pubis.

(b) It covers both the surfaces of uterus.

(c) It continues from anteroinferior surface of uterus to the anterior vaginal fornix before reflecting over the superior surface of urinary bladder to form uterovesical pouch.

(d) It is reflected from front of rectum to the posterior vaginal fornix and uterus forming rectouterine pouch (of Douglas).

(e) Rectouterine pouch is the most dependant part in the pelvis during supine posture.

360. Pelvic vessels

(a) Pelvis is supplied by the branches arising from internal iliac artery.

(b) There are 3 parietal (inferior gluteal, internal pudendal and obturator) and 3 visceral (vesical, middle rectal and inferior rectal) branches arising from anterior division of internal iliac artery.

(c) Posterior division of internal iliac artery provides only 3 parietal branches (iliolumbar, superior gluteal and lateral sacral).

(d) Veins derived from pelvis ultimately drain into internal iliac vein.

(e) Pelvic veins show tendency to form plexuses in relation to viscera (rectal, uterine, prostatic and vesical).

361. Nerves of the pelvis

(a) These are of 4 kinds—2 autonomic (sacral sympathetic trunk and pelvic plexus) and 2 somatic (sacral plexus and obturator nerve).

(b) Sacral plexus is formed by ventral rami of upper 4 sacral nerves.

(c) Three branches (nerve to obturator internus, nerve to quadratus femoris and tibial component of sciatic nerve) arise from anterior division of sacral plexus.

(d) Three branches (2 gluteal nerves and 1 common peroneal component of sciatic nerve) appear from posterior divisions of sacral plexus.

(e) Direct branches from sacral nerves are – nerve to piriformis, perforating cutaneous nerve, posterior cutaneous nerve of thigh, pelvic splanchnic nerves, pudendal nerve and perineal branch of S_4 (formula of P).

362. Urinary bladder–I

(a) It is endodermal in origin except trigone which is mesodermal.

(b) Its capacity is about 280 ml which initiates reflex micturition.

(c) The pain is felt when the volume of fluid in it is more than 350 ml.

(d) It is tetrahedral in shape when empty.

(e) It has borders – 2 lateral, 1 anterior, 1 posterior; surfaces – 2 inferolateral, 1 superior; base, apex and neck.

363. Urinary bladder–II

(a) Trigone is a smooth triangular area in the upper part of the interior of the base.

(b) Each angle of the trigone is marked by an orifice (2 ureteric and 1 internal urethral).

(c) Its superior (intestine), inferolateral (obturator internus and levator ani) and anterior (cave of Retzius) relations are identical in two sexes.

(d) Posterior surface (base) is related to seminal vesicle, vas deferens and rectum in male while vagina and cervix in female.

(e) It is supported by ligaments (median umbilical, lateral and pubovesical).

364. Urinary bladder–III

(a) It is supplied by vesical (superior and inferior) branches of internal iliac and pubic branches of inferior epigastric arteries.

(b) It is drained by prostatic-vesical venous plexus.

(c) Its lymphatics accompany the blood vessels and drain into internal and external iliac lymph nodes.

(d) Its efferent nerve fibres are both sympathetic (T_{12}–L_2) and parasympathetic (S_2–S_4) in nature while its afferent fibres run mainly along the parasympathetic part.

(e) Micturition is a reflex phenomenon occurring at the level of spinal segments T_{12}–L_2.

365. Prostate–I

(a) It is a pyramidal (base up, apex down) fibromuscular gland located between the neck of urinary bladder and urogenital diaphragm.

(b) Its length (base to apex) is about 6 cm.

(c) It is related anteriorly with the cave of Retzius and pubo-prostatic ligament, laterally with levator ani and posteriorly with fascia of Denonvillier and rectum.

(d) It is surrounded by true and false capsules with prostatic venous plexus between the two.

(e) It has 5 lobes – 1 anterior, 1 median, 1 posterior and 2 lateral.

366. Prostate–II

(a) Prostatic urethra is 3 cm in length and relatively widest.

(b) Utriculus musculinus, a depression in the middle of urethral crest, is homologous of uterus in female.

(c) It is supplied by inferior vesical and middle rectal arteries.

(d) Benign prostatic hypertrophy usually involves its main glands while malignancy occurs in mucous and submucous glands.

(e) In cases of its malignancy, per rectal examination reveals lack of posterior midline groove in it and fixation of rectal wall over it.

367. Rectum–I

(a) It extends from 3rd sacral vertebra to anorectal junction located 5 cm anteroinferior to tip of coccyx.

(b) It measures about 12 cm in length, of which proximal 7 cm lies over sacrum and coccyx and distal 5 cm rests over anococcygeal raphe.

(c) It has three lateral convexities, upper and lower are facing towards right side while middle one is directed to left.

(d) Peritoneum covers its upper one-third (anterior and lateral) and middle one-third (anterior) only, while lower one-third is devoid of peritoneal covering.

(e) Its upper part is named as rectal ampulla.

368. Rectum–II

(a) It is supported by fascia of Waldeyer, lateral ligament of rectum, pelvic peritoneum and pelvic diaphragm.

(b) Superior and middle rectal and median sacral arteries supply it, of which the former provides three branches corresponding with 4, 7, and 11 o'clock positions in lithotomy posture.

(c) It is drained by superior and middle rectal veins which are tributaries of internal iliac and inferior mesenteric veins respectively.

(d) Its lymphatics drain into periaortic, internal iliac and sacral lymph nodes.

(e) Its sympathetic (T_{12}–L_2) and parasympathetic (S_2–S_4) fibres are derived from pelvic plexus.

369. Anal canal–I

(a) It makes a 90° bend at anorectal junction and runs for about 3 cm to end into anus.

(b) Anorectal junction is marked by puborectalis sling.

(c) Its upper two-thirds is derived from cloaca while lower one-third originates from anal pit.

(d) Its lateral (ischiorectal fossa) and posterior (anococcygeal body and tip of coccyx) relations are same in two sexes.

(e) It is related anteriorly to prostate and perineal body in male while vagina and perineal body in female.

370. Anal canal–II

(a) Circular and longitudinal muscle coats of rectum continue into the anal canal's upper two-thirds as internal anal sphincter and conjoint longitudinal layer, respectively.

(b) Union of lower ends of anal columns in the upper part of anal canal forms annulus haemorrhoidalis which corresponds with the surgeon's dentate line.

(c) A relatively avascular ring (Hilton's white line) lies below the dentate line and marks the beginning of stratified squamous epithelium.

(d) Mucosa of the upper two-thirds of anal canal is supplied by the same nerves and vessels which are meant for rectum.

(e) Mucosa of the lower one-third of anal canal is supplied by somatic nerve (inferior rectal branch of internal pudendal nerve) and therefore is less sensitive.

371. Ovary–I

(a) It is located in the ovarian fossa bounded anteriorly by superior vesical artery and posteriorly by internal iliac artery and ureter.

(b) Its length, width and thickness are about 3, 1.5 and 1 cm, respectively.

(c) It has 2 extremities (upper and lower), 2 borders (anterior and posterior) and 2 surfaces (medial and lateral).

(d) It is connected with posterior leaf of broad ligament of uterus by mesovasium.

(e) Its upper and lower poles are connected with suspensory ligament and ligament of ovary, respectively.

372. Ovary–II

(a) Its germ cells are endodermal in origin and derived from the wall of yolk sac during development.

(b) It is supplied by ovarian artery derived from aorta reminding its abdominal development.

(c) Ovarian vein is a tributary of right renal vein on the right and inferior vena cava on the left side.

(d) Ovarian lymphatics drain into lateral aortic lymph nodes near the origin of ovarian artery explaining an abdominal lump in cases of ovarian malignancy.

(e) Its sympathetic fibres (T_{10}–L_2) are vasomotor in nature and explain the referred pain to it in cases of appendicitis and renal colic.

373. Uterus–I

(a) It is a thick-walled muscular organ located between the urinary bladder and rectum.

(b) It weighs about 100 g.

(c) Its height, width and thickness are 7.5 (body–5 cm, cervix– 2.5 cm), 5 and 2.5 cm, respectively.

(d) Endometrium is special name given to its mucosa which is renamed as decidua during pregnancy.

(e) Normal uterus is anteflexed (forward bending of the body over cervix) and anteverted (forward bending of the whole uterus over vagina).

374. Uterus–II

(a) Its lumen is slit-like in transverse section but triangular and fusiform in the regions of body and cervix respectively in section parallel to its surfaces.

(b) The peritoneum, after covering its anterior and posterior surfaces, continues beyond its lateral margin as broad ligament of uterus.

(c) Three main ligaments supporting it are suspensory ligament, broad ligament and ligament of ovary.

(d) Its blood supply is derived from internal iliac vessels.

(e) All the lymphatics drain into lateral aortic and external and internal iliac lymph nodes except some of them from fundus which reach the superficial inguinal group along its round ligament.

375. Fallopian tube

(a) It is located in the upper free margin of broad ligament of uterus.

(b) It is divisible into intramural, isthmus (medial one-third), ampulla (lateral two-thirds) and infundibulum.

(c) It measures about 10. cm in length.

(d) Its medial one-third is supplied by uterine artery while lateral two-thirds by ovarian artery.

(e) Its lumen shows characteristically excessive mucosal foldings.

376. Vagina

(a) It is located between the rectum and anal canal posteriorly and urinary bladder and urethra anteriorly.

(b) The lengths of its anterior and posterior walls are 9 and 7.5 cm, respectively.

(c) In transverse section, its lumen is—circular in upper one-third, slit like in the middle one-third and H-shaped in the lower one-third.

(d) It is supplied by uterine artery in its upper part and vaginal artery in its lower part, both emerging from internal iliac artery.

(e) Lymphatics from its upper part drain into internal iliac lymph nodes while those from its lower part enter the superficial inguinal lymph nodes.

377. Ischiorectal fossa

(a) It is a wedge-shaped space on each side of anal canal with its edge upwards and base downwards.

(b) Its lateral wall is formed by ischiopubic ramus and fascia over obturator internus.

(c) Its medial wall is formed by external anal sphincters and inferior fascia of pelvic diaphragm.

(d) Perianal fascia divides this fossa into deep (ischiorectal space) and superficial (perianal space) parts.

(e) Abscess in the perianal space is very painful due to its compartmentalization by complete septa into small fat loculi.

378. Pudendal (Alcock's) canal

(a) It is located in the lateral wall of ischiorectal fossa over the obturator fascia.

(b) It connects the lesser sciatic foramen with the posterior border of perineal membrane.

(c) It is contributed by the perianal fascia which thickens and splits to enclose the pudendal nerve and internal pudendal vessels, i.e. its contents.

(d) Both, pudendal nerve and internal pudendal artery, provide a perineal branch in its posterior part.

(e) In case of pudendal block, the local anaesthetic solution is infiltrated around pudendal nerve proximal to its entry into the pudendal canal.

379. Female external genital organs

(a) The mons pubis is rounded eminence in front of pubic symphysis.

(b) Labia majora are longitudinal cutaneous folds with excessive fat, on each side of pudendal cleft.

(c) Labia minora are two small cutaneous folds devoid of fat, between labia majora.

(d) Labia minora splits anteriorly to enclose the clitoris which is homologous of penis.

(e) In the vestibule (area between labia minora) is situated external urethral orifice 5 cm behind the clitoris.

380. Penis

(a) It consists of an attached part, called as root and a free part known as body.

(b) Its root is comprised of two crura related to ischiopubic ramus on each side and one median bulb.

(c) Corpus cavernosus, erectile tissue in each crus, continues on the dorsolateral aspect of body while corpus spongiosum of bulb occupies the ventral midline of the body.

(d) It is supported by ligamentum frondosum (from linea alba to penis) and suspensory ligament (from pubic symphysis to penis).

(e) Its erection is a sympathetic phenomenon while ejaculation is a parasympathetic phenomenon.

381. Perineum

(a) It is part of pelvic outlet between pelvic diaphragm and perineal membrane.

(b) It is divisible into smaller anterior urogenital triangle and larger posterior anal triangle by a line between anterior ends of ischial tuberosities.

(c) The skin of anal triangle is supplied by inferior rectal nerve (S_3, S_4) perineal branch of S_4 and coccygeal plexus (S_5).

(d) Anterior axial line marks the junction of anterior one-third with the posterior two-thirds of scrotum or labium majus.

(e) The skin of urogenital triangle anterior to anterior axial line is supplied by ilioinguinal nerve while posterior to this line is innervated by perineal branches of posterior cutaneous nerve of thigh and pudendal nerve.

382. Pudendal nerve

(a) It emerges from the sacral plexus (S_2–S_4) in the pelvis.

(b) It crosses the tip of sacrospinous ligament medial to internal pudendal artery during its course from greater sciatic foramen to lesser sciatic foramen.

(c) Its inferior rectal nerve appearing in the posterior part of Alcock's canal, first ascends over the obturator fascia and then runs medially under the pelvic diaphragm to reach the anal canal.

(d) Inferior rectal branch is purely cutaneous in the region of anal triangle.

(e) It terminates into perineal nerve and dorsal nerve of penis (clitoris) which enter the superficial and deep perineal pouches, respectively.

383. Internal pudendal artery

(a) It is a parietal branch arising from the posterior division of internal iliac artery.

(b) It crosses the tip of ischial spine between nerve to obturator internus and pudendal nerve during its course from greater sciatic foramen to lesser sciatic foramen.

(c) Its 1st branch is inferior rectal artery which accompanies inferior rectal nerve and never supplies rectum.

(d) Its 2nd set of branches (transverse perineal and scrotal or labial) appear near the posterior margin of perineal membrane.

(e) It terminates by dividing into branches in the deep perineal pouch to supply penis (clitoris).

384. Deep perineal pouch–I

   (a) Its roof is formed by inferior fascia of pelvic diaphragm also called superior fascia of urogenital diaphragm.

   (b) Perineal membrane lies in its floor.

   (c) Its muscles, nerves and vessels together constitute the urogenital diaphragm.

   (d) The sphincter urethrae in male consist of transversely lying looped muscle fibres and anteroposteriorly situated straight fibres in relation to urethra.

   (e) The sphincter urethrae in female consist of circular fibres around urethra and anteroposterior fibres on each side of latter.

385. Deep perineal pouch–II

   (a) Deep transversus perinei extends from corresponding ischiopubic rami to perineal body to which it provides support.

   (b) Its two muscles (sphincter urethrae and deep transversus perinei) receive innervation from the dorsal nerve of penis (clitoris).

   (c) Bulbourethral glands of Cowper are located on each side of urethra in this pouch in male.

   (d) Its nerve is dorsal nerve of penis (clitoris), one of the terminal branches of pudendal nerve.

   (e) Its arteries are terminal branches of internal pudendal artery meant for penis (clitoris).

386. Perineal membrane

   (a) It bridges the ischiopubic rami of the two sides and has free anterior and posterior (transverse perineal ligament) margins.

   (b) Between the transverse perineal ligament and inferior pubic ligament is the passage for deep dorsal vein of penis and dorsal nerve of penis in male.

   (c) It is traversed by urethra and duct of Cowper's gland in male while urethra and vagina in female.

   (d) Scrotal (labial) nerve and artery pierce this membrane near its posterior margin.

(e) Arteries of penis (deep artery, dorsal artery, artery of bulb) or clitoris (deep artery, dorsal artery) pierce the membrane before reaching the genitalia.

387. Superficial perineal pouch–I

(a) Its roof is formed by perineal membrane.

(b) Its floor is formed by fascia of Colles (continuation of fascia of Scarpa from abdomen).

(c) It lodges crura of penis (crura of clitoris in female) and bulb of penis (bulb of vestibule in female).

(d) Greater vestibular gland is located in this space on each side, lateral to bulb of vestibule in female.

(e) In male the urethra enters the bulb and continues into the penis while in female the space is traversed by urethra and vagina which open on the surface.

388. Superficial perineal pouch–II

(a) It lodges superficial transversus perinei which runs transversely from ischiopubic rami to perineal body.

(b) Ischiocavernosus extends from the ischial tuberosity to the crus of penis or clitoris.

(c) In male, the bulbocavernosus extends laterally to the bulb and body of penis from perineal body and midline raphe while in female it runs forwards from perineal body to clitoris on each side of vagina.

(d) The perineal branch of pudendal nerve enters this pouch and splits into muscular and scrotal (labial) branches.

(e) No branch of internal pudendal artery is visibly running a course in this pouch as all the branches enter the penis (clitoris) directly after piercing the perineal membrane.

389. Perineal body

(a) It is a fibromuscular mass anterior to anal canal.

(b) It extends from the pelvic diaphragm to the level of perineal membrane.

(c) Anteriorly, it is related with the vagina in female and apex of prostate, membranous urethra and bulb of penis in male.

(d) Its muscular fibres are derived from both transversus perinei (superficial and deep), superficial external anal sphincter, puboprostaticus (pubovaginalis in female) and bulbo-cavernosus.

(e) It is of great obstetrical importance due to its important role in support of pelvic organs and its occasional damage during parturition.

KEY CHART

1. (c)	2. (c)	3. (a)	4. (e)	5. (a)
6. (e)	7. (b)	8. (a)	9. (b)	10. (c)
11. (e)	12. (d)	13. (c)	14. (e)	15. (d)
16. (a)	17. (b)	18. (c)	19. (c)	20. (c)
21. (b)	22. (c)	23. (a)	24. (e)	25. (a)
26. (b)	27. (c)	28. (e)	29. (d)	30. (c)
31. (c)	32. (e)	33. (a)	34. (c)	35. (d)
36. (c)	37. (b)	38. (c)	39. (a)	40. (e)
41. (c)	42. (c)	43. (d)	44. (e)	45. (b)
46. (a)	47. (a)	48. (c)	49. (c)	50. (e)
51. (a)	52. (d)	53. (d)	54. (b)	55. (c)
56. (a)	57. (d)	58. (d)	59. (b)	60. (c)
61. (e)	62. (a)	63. (e)	64. (a)	65. (e)
66. (d)	67. (b)	68. (e)	69. (c)	70. (c)
71. (a)	72. (b)	73. (b)	74. (c)	75. (e)
76. (e)	77. (e)	78. (a)	79. (d)	80. (e)
81. (b)	82. (b)	83. (d)	84. (a)	85. (d)
86. (a)	87. (d)	88. (e)	89. (c)	90. (b)
91. (b)	92. (c)	93. (d)	94. (e)	95. (d)
96. (b)	97. (a)	98. (b)	99. (d)	100. (e)
101. (a)	102. (e)	103. (e)	104. (d)	105. (b)
106. (a)	107. (a)	108. (b)	109. (d)	110. (c)
111. (c)	112. (a)	113. (e)	114. (d)	115. (d)
116. (d)	117. (e)	118. (b)	119. (c)	120. (e)
121. (d)	122. (d)	123. (b)	124. (c)	125. (d)
126. (e)	127. (c)	128. (c)	129. (b)	130. (b)
131. (a)	132. (d)	133. (d)	134. (d)	135. (b)
136. (b)	137. (b)	138. (c)	139. (c)	140. (c)
141. (a)	142. (d)	143. (b)	144. (e)	145. (b)

146. (a)	147. (d)	148. (e)	149. (c)	150. (e)
151. (e)	152. (c)	153. (c)	154. (c)	155. (c)
156. (b)	157. (d)	158. (d)	159. (e)	160. (c)
161. (c)	162. (c)	163. (a)	164. (e)	165. (c)
166. (e)	167. (e)	168. (d)	169. (c)	170. (e)
171. (d)	172. (d)	173. (c)	174. (e)	175. (d)
176. (b)	177. (e)	178. (b)	179. (e)	180. (a)
181. (e)	182. (c)	183. (d)	184. (b)	185. (b)
186. (b)	187. (a)	188. (b)	189. (b)	190. (e)
191. (d)	192. (b)	193. (e)	194. (c)	195. (d)
196. (b)	197. (a)	198. (e)	199. (a)	200. (b)
201. (d)	202. (e)	203. (a)	204. (d)	205. (a)
206. (b)	207. (c)	208. (b)	209. (a)	210. (b)
211. (d)	212. (a)	213. (d)	214. (e)	215. (c)
216. (a)	217. (c)	218. (b)	219. (e)	220. (c)
221. (d)	222. (d)	223. (e)	224. (a)	225. (a)
226. (c)	227. (a)	228. (b)	229. (c)	230. (d)
231. (d)	232. (a)	233. (d)	234. (a)	235. (c)
236. (b)	237. (c)	238. (d)	239. (a)	240. (e)
241. (b)	242. (d)	243. (b)	244. (e)	245. (c)
246. (a)	247. (c)	248. (b)	249. (c)	250. (e)
251. (e)	252. (c)	253. (a)	254. (d)	255. (e)
256. (c)	257. (b)	258. (a)	259. (c)	260. (b)
261. (a)	262. (c)	263. (e)	264. (e)	265. (a)
266. (d)	267. (b)	268. (c)	269. (d)	270. (a)
271. (a)	272. (b)	273. (c)	274. (d)	275. (e)
276. (c)	277. (a)	278. (b)	279. (d)	280. (e)
281. (d)	282. (b)	283. (d)	284. (a)	285. (e)
286. (c)	287. (a)	288. (c)	289. (b)	290. (d)
291. (a)	292. (d)	293. (c)	294. (b)	295. (b)
296. (a)	297. (d)	298. (c)	299. (b)	300. (a)

301. (e)	302. (a)	303. (a)	304. (d)	305. (c)
306. (b)	307. (b)	308. (a)	309. (e)	310. (c)
311. (d)	312. (b)	313. (c)	314. (d)	315. (e)
316. (b)	317. (a)	318. (b)	319. (c)	320. (c)
321. (a)	322. (e)	323. (e)	324. (b)	325. (a)
326. (d)	327. (d)	328. (a)	329. (b)	330. (c)
331. (d)	332. (c)	333. (a)	334. (c)	335. (b)
336. (e)	337. (d)	338. (e)	339. (c)	340. (e)
341. (a)	342. (c)	343. (b)	344. (c)	345. (a)
346. (d)	347. (e)	348. (b)	349. (c)	350. (a)
351. (b)	352. (e)	353. (b)	354. (c)	355. (e)
356. (e)	357. (c)	358. (b)	359. (c)	360. (b)
361. (b)	362. (c)	363. (a)	364. (e)	365. (b)
366. (d)	367. (e)	368. (c)	369. (e)	370. (e)
371. (a)	372. (c)	373. (b)	374. (c)	375. (d)
376. (b)	377. (b)	378. (d)	379. (e)	380. (e)
381. (a)	382. (d)	383. (a)	384. (c)	385. (b)
386. (a)	387. (d)	388. (e)	389. (b)	

KEY WITH CORRECT STATEMENTS

1. (c) The mandible is second to clavicle to ossify.

2. (c) The jugular arch connecting the two anterior jugular veins lies above the jugular notch.

3. (a) The skin above the level of sternal angle of Louis is supplied by the supraclavicular nerves (C_3, C_4).

4. (e) Most of lymphatics from breast drain into axillary lymph nodes.

5. (a) The clavipectoral fascia strengthens the anterior wall of axilla.

6. (e) The axillary tail (of Spence) of breast pierces the floor to enter the axilla.

7. (b) The relations of cords of brachial plexus to the 2nd part of axillary artery are indicated by their names.

8. (a) The divisions of brachial plexus lie behind the clavicle.

9. (b) In the upper part of body, medial branches, while in the lower part, lateral branches of the dorsal rami give rise to cutaneous twigs.

10. (c) The motor supply of trapezius is derived from the accessory spinal nerve, while its sensory (proprioceptive) supply comes from 3rd and 4th cervical ventral rami.

11. (e) The long heads of biceps brachii and triceps arise from supraglenoid and infraglenoid tubercles of scapula, respectively.

12. (d) The most important stabilizing factor during scapular movements at acromioclavicular joint is coracoclavicular ligament.

13. (c) The innervation of latissimus dorsi is derived from thoracodorsal nerve.

14. (e) The back of lateral epicondyle of humerus provides attachment to the anconeus.

15. (d) The Colles' fracture involves the lower end of the radius.

16. (a) The posterior border of the ulna is subcutaneous and gives attachment to the deep fascia of forearm.

17. (b) Swelling and tenderness in anatomical snuffbox indicate fracture of scaphoid.

18. (c)   The cephalic vein drains into the axillary vein.

19. (c)   The supratrochlear lymph nodes receive lymphatics from the medial fingers.

20. (c)   The dorsal aspects of distal parts of the lateral three and half digits are innervated by the median nerve.

21. (b)   There is quite considerable overlapping between the continuous adjacent dermatomes.

22. (c)   The deep fascia of the forearm is firmly fixed to the posterior border of the ulna.

23. (a)   The acromial part of the deltoid is multipennate in nature.

24. (e)   The supraspinatus is innervated by the suprascapular branch of upper trunk of brachial plexus.

25. (a)   The articular disc, often present inside the acromioclavicular joint, is rarely a complete one.

26. (b)   The rotator cuff muscles form the most important stabilizing factor of the shoulder joint

27. (c)   Besides the two muscles (deltoid and teres minor), the axillary nerve also supplies the skin (over lower part of deltoid) and the joint (shoulder).

28. (e)   The circumflex scapular artery is a branch of subscapular artery.

29. (d)   The biceps brachii is one of the muscles involved in Erb - Duchenne paralysis.

30. (c)   In the cubital fossa, the brachial artery is sandwiched between the biceps tendon and the median nerve.

31. (c)   After supplying muscles of flexor compartment of arm, the musculocutaneous nerve continues as lateral cutaneous nerve of forearm.

32. (e)   The ulnar nerve gives off no muscular branch in the arm.

33. (a)   The median nerve is formed, by the union of its medial and lateral roots, on the lateral aspect of 3rd part of the axillary artery.

34. (c)   The brachial artery terminates at the level of neck of radius by dividing into radial and ulnar arteries.

35. (d)   Separate branches of the radial nerve innervate the three heads of the triceps.

36. (c) The radial nerve also runs a course in the flexor compartment of the distal arm, in addition to its course in the extensor compartment of the proximal arm.

37. (b) Flexor digitorum superficialis lies deep to the other four muscles of the superficial group, i.e. pronator teres, flexor carpi radialis, palmaris longus and flexor carpi ulnaris.

38. (c) Distally, the palmar aponeurosis divides into four slips, one for each of the medial four digits.

39. (a) The superficial palmar arch is formed by continuation of the ulnar artery in hand.

40. (e) Carpal tunnel syndrome is produced by compression of the median nerve deep to the flexor retinaculum.

41. (c) The radial bursa is the synovial sheath for tendon of flexor pollicis longus.

42. (c) Anterior interosseous artery also enters the extensor compartment of the forearm.

43. (d) The median nerve injury in forearm differs from the carpal tunnel syndrome, as in the latter condition cutaneous sensation over thenar eminence remains intact.

44. (e) Injury to the ulnar nerve leads to "claw hand" deformity, in which there is extension at metacarpophalangeal joints and flexion at interphalangeal joints.

45. (b) Tenosynovitis in the little finger is likely to involve midpalmar space.

46. (a) The thenar eminence is produced by abductor pollicis brevis, flexor pollicis brevis and opponens pollicis only.

47. (a) In addition to abductor, flexor and opponens digiti minimi, the palmaris brevis is also included in the hypothenar eminence muscles.

48. (c) Three palmar metacarpal arteries arise directly from the deep palmar arch and join the corresponding common palmar digital arteries, branches of the superficial palmar arch.

49. (c) The tendon of extensor pollicis longus grooves the dorsal tubercle (of Lister) of radius on its medial aspect.

50. (e) The tendon of extensor carpi ulnaris passes through the most medial of the compartments under the extensor retinaculum.

51. (a) The palmar interossei adduct while the dorsal interossei abduct the digits.

52. (d) The elbow and superior radioulnar joints share a common joint cavity.

53. (d) Forceful separation of the radial head from the capitulum of humerus, in adult individuals, is prevented mainly by the anular ligament.

54. (b) Because of the higher level of the ulnar styloid process, the range of adduction at wrist is greater than that of abduction.

55. (c) The mesenchymal core of the limb is derived from the somatopleuric mesoderm.

56. (a) Three constituents of the hip bone, ilium, ischium and pubis, meet at acetabulum to form a "Y" shaped (triradiate) junction.

57. (d) The vastus intermedius is attached to front and lateral surface of the femoral shaft.

58. (d) The anterior border of tibia provides attachment to deep fascia of leg, while the interosseous membrane is attached to its interosseous (lateral) border.

59. (b) The appearance of the secondary centre and its fusion with the shaft take place later at its upper end than at its lower end

60. (c) The sustentaculum tali is a projection from the medial aspect of the calcaneus.

61. (e) Most of the cutaneous nerves for the front of thigh are derived from anterior division of the femoral nerve.

62. (a) Most of the superficial lymphatics of lower limb drain into vertical chain of the superficial inguinal lymph nodes.

63. (e) Incompetent valves in communicating veins present in lower limb result into flow of blood from deep to superficial and therefore lead to varicose veins.

64. (a) Iliotibial tract is a thickened band on the lateral aspect of the fascia lata.

65. (e) The intermediate part of femoral sheath is occupied by femoral vein while in its lateral part lie femoral artery and femoral branch of genitofemoral nerve.

66. (d) The femoral artery can be most effectively compressed against the head of the femur.

67. (b) The femoral nerve is derived from dorsal divisions of the ventral rami of 2nd, 3rd and 4th lumbar nerves.

68. (e) The sartorius causes flexion of leg, and flexion, abduction and lateral rotation of thigh (cross-legged or tailor's posture).

69. (c) In addition to adduction, the three adductors also cause medial rotation of the thigh.

70. (c) The femoral vessels, saphenous nerve and nerve to vastus medialis constitute the contents of the adductor canal.

71. (a) The profunda femoris artery arises from the femoral artery 3.5 cm below the inguinal ligament.

72. (b) The obturator nerve terminates into its anterior and posterior divisions in the pelvis, before entering the thigh.

73. (b) Upper lateral quadrant is the most suitable site for the intramuscular injections in the gluteal region.

74. (c) The superior gemellus is supplied by nerve to obturator internus, while the inferior gemellus is innervated by nerve to quadratus femoris.

75. (e) The nerve to obturator internus lies most laterally while entering the lesser sciatic foramen along with the pudendal nerve and internal pudendal vessels.

76. (e) The companion artery of sciatic nerve (axial artery) springs from the inferior gluteal artery.

77. (e) The short head of biceps femoris is not included in hamstring group of muscles.

78. (a) The root value of sciatic nerve is L_4, L_5, S_1-S_3.

79. (d) The branches from the lower end of peroneal artery contribute to the lateral malleolar arterial network.

80. (e) The upper medial boundary of the popliteal fossa is formed by the semimembranosus and semitendinosus.

81. (b) The popliteal artery is the deepest of all the contents of the popliteal fossa.

82. (b) The sural nerve supplies lower lateral part of the posterior aspect of the leg.

83. (d) Distal limb of the V-shaped inferior extensor retinaculum blends medially with the plantar aponeurosis.

84. (a) All the muscles of the extensor compartment of leg arise from the fibula except the tibialis anterior, which originates from the tibia.

85. (d) The deep peroneal nerve lies lateral to the anterior tibial artery underneath the superior extensor retinaculum.

86. (a) Only the peronei longus and brevis constitute the peroneal compartment muscles.

87. (d) The strength of gastrocnemius is less while its range of movement is more than that of the soleus.

88. (e) The back of medial malleolus is grooved by the tendon of tibialis posterior.

89. (c) The posterior tibial artery runs medial to the tibial nerve under the flexor retinaculum to enter the sole.

90. (b) In addition to supplying extensor digitorum brevis, deep peroneal nerve also innervates the skin of 1st inter digital cleft and adjacent sides of 1st and 2nd toes.

91. (b) The skin of the sole is very thick due to the thickened epidermis.

92. (c) The flexor digitorum brevis and abductor hallucis are supplied by medial plantar nerve.

93. (d) The medial most lumbrical is supplied by the medial plantar nerve while the remaining three lumbricals are innervated by the lateral plantar nerve.

94. (e) The flexor hallucis brevis is a unique muscle in the sense that it has got dual insertion.

95. (d) Both the 1st and 2nd dorsal interossei act on the 2nd toe.

96. (b) The medial plantar nerve supplies the four muscles in total, two in the 1st (abductor hallucis and flexor digitorum brevis), and one each in 2nd (first lumbrical) and 3rd (flexor hallucis brevis) muscular layers of the sole.

97. (a) The proximal part of the lateral plantar nerve runs obliquely lateralwards between 1st and 2nd muscular layers of the sole.

98. (b) The plantar arch is formed by the distal curved part of the lateral plantar artery.

99. (d) The capacity of the hip joint cavity is maximum when the thigh is flexed, abducted and laterally rotated, the posture

preferably adopted by the patients suffering from painful inflammatory conditions of this joint.

100. (e) Medial meniscus is commonly crushed between femur and tibia.

101. (a) The superior tibiofibular joint is a plane type of synovial joint.

102. (e) The plantar flexion is accompanied by inversion while the dorsiflexion by eversion.

103. (e) The interphalangeal joints are hinge type of synovial joints.

104. (d) When the arches of foot are collapsed, the condition is called "flat foot" (pes planus).

105. (b) The superior aperture of thorax is narrower than its inferior one.

106. (a) All the sternocostal joints are of the synovial type, except the 1st one which is a primary cartilaginous joint (synchondrosis).

107. (a) First rib is the most curved rib.

108. (b) The medial part of inner surface of the 12th rib is related to the costal pleura.

109. (d) The floor of the costal groove gives attachment to the internal intercostal.

110. (c) Of all the thoracic vertebrae, the 3rd one has got the smallest body.

111. (c) The plane of the superior aperture of thorax has an obliquity of about 45 degrees.

112. (a) The pump handle movement increases the anteroposterior diameter of the thorax.

113. (e) The inferior aperture of the thorax is wider transversely than anteroposteriorly.

114. (d) The 3rd (deepest) layer of the intercostal muscles consists of subcostalis and transversus thoracis (sternocostalis), in addition to intercostalis intimus.

115. (d) To avoid injury to the intercostal nerve, a clinician should introduce the needle near the upper border of the rib.

116. (d) Internal thoracic artery is ligated preferably in the 2nd intercostal space.

117. (e) Both hemiazygos and accessory hemiazygos veins cross the body of 8th thoracic vertebra to enter the azygos vein.

118. (b) The superior mediastinum is separated from the inferior one by a plane passing between 4th and 5th thoracic vertebrae.

119. (c) Visceral pleura is not sensitive to pain.

120. (e) The root of the lung is arched by azygos vein on the right side, and arch of aorta on the left side.

121. (d) Thoracic sympathetic ganglia are connected to the ventral rami of corresponding spinal nerves by both grey and white rami communicantes.

122. (d) The vena azygos is provided with only a few incompetent valves.

123. (b) The phrenic nerve descends usually in front of the subclavian artery.

124. (c) Anomalous azygos lobe may be present in the right lung.

125. (d) A "subapical" segment is present in the lower lobe of the right lung in more than 50 % of the individuals.

126. (e) The main bronchial vessels run on the dorsal aspect of the extrapulmonary bronchi.

127. (c) The efferents of tracheobronchial lymph nodes enter into bronchomediastinal trunks.

128. (c) The thymus is derived from the 3rd pharyngeal pouch (endodermal).

129. (b) The base of the fibrous pericardium, which faces inferiorly does not correspond with the base of the heart, which is directed posteriorly.

130. (b) The right border of the heart lies about 1.2 cm lateral to the right sternal margin.

131. (a) The left coronary artery is commonly larger in diameter than the right one.

132. (d) The oblique vein of left atrium (of Marshall) is the remnant of distal part of the left common cardinal vein.

133. (d) The afferents for cardiac pain travel in all the sympathetic cardiac nerves except the superior cervical one.

134. (d) The opening of the coronary sinus lies between right atrioventricular orifice and opening of the inferior vena cava.

135. (b) The superior vena cava is formed by the union of two brachiocephalic veins opposite the lower border of right 1st

costal cartilage and enters the right atrium at the level of upper border of right 3rd costal cartilage.

136. (b) The thickness of wall of the right ventricle is one-third of the left ventricular wall.

137. (b) The pulmonary trunk lies first in front and then to the left of the ascending aorta.

138. (c) The aortic vestibule is mainly elastic in nature and facilitates the propulsion of blood by its elastic recoil.

139. (c) The two (right and left) coronary arteries arise from the aortic sinuses of the ascending aorta.

140. (c) Internal thoracic, vertebral, inferior thyroid and 1st posterior (highest) intercostal veins are the tributaries of corresponding brachiocephalic vein, in addition to its main tributaries, i.e. internal jugular and subclavian veins.

141. (a) The arch of aorta arches over the root of the left lung behind the lower half of the manubrium sterni.

142. (d) The pulmonary arteries carry deoxygenated blood and supply nutrition to the alveoli only.

143. (b) The smooth part of the left atrium develops by incorporation of the pulmonary veins, while its rough part is derived from the primitive atrium.

144. (e) The Purkinje fibres are subendocardial in position.

145. (b) The C-shaped tracheal rings of hyaline cartilage occupy the anterior aspect and the sides of the trachea leaving a gap posteriorly, which is filled by the muscle trachealis.

146. (a) The preganglionic sympathetic neurons for the cardiac plexus are located in the intermediolateral column of the upper 5 thoracic segments of the spinal cord.

147. (d) The vagi descend and break up behind the corresponding roots of the lungs to form pulmonary plexuses along with the sympathetic twigs from 2nd, 3rd and 4th thoracic sympathetic ganglia.

148. (e) The sympathetic fibres of the pulmonary plexus are bronchodilator and vasoconstrictor in nature.

149. (c) The oesophagus does show curvatures, both in sagittal (conforming to the vertebral curvatures) and coronal (convex leftward superiorly and rightward inferiorly) planes.

150. (e) The thoracic duct does have numerous valves.

151. (e) In primary pulmonary tuberculosis, the tracheobronchial group of lymph nodes are invariably involved.

152. (c) All the sternocostal joints from 2nd to 7th are of synovial type with a single joint cavity except the 2nd one, which has double cavities.

153. (c) The bucket handle movement is facilitated by the flat articular surfaces of the costotransverse joints of lower (7th to 10th) ribs.

154. (c) Three primary cerebral vesicles; prosencephalon, mesencephalon and rhombencephalon grow to form the forebrain, midbrain and hindbrain, respectively.

155. (c) The dendrites differ from the axons due to the presence of branching and Nissl substance.

156. (b) The fibrous astrocytes are present mainly in the white matter.

157. (d) The forebrain consists of the two cerebral hemispheres as well as the diencephalon.

158. (d) The dura mater is mesodermal in origin.

159. (e) The arachnoid mater and the dura mater are usually pierced by the cranial nerves at the same points.

160. (c) The volume of the cerebrospinal fluid is greatly increased from the normal, in cases of the hydrocephalus.

161. (c) The pia mater is adherent to the brain surfaces and dips into the sulci.

162. (c) The superficial middle cerebral vein joins the cavernous sinus.

163. (a) The basal vein is formed by the union of anterior cerebral, striate and deep middle cerebral veins.

164. (e) In many cases, the collateral circulation in circle of Willis is not adequate enough to prevent the hemiplegia of the opposite side, if one internal carotid artery is suddenly blocked.

165. (c) Somatic motor and somatic sensory areas are supplied by both anterior and middle cerebral arteries.

166. (e) The Charcot's artery (of cerebral haemorrhage), most commonly involved in the cerebrovascular accidents, is usually the largest of all lateral striate central arteries.

167. (e) Thrombosis in the posterior inferior cerebellar artery is responsible for the lateral medullary (Wallenberg) syndrome.

168. (d) V, VII, VIII, IX, X cranial nerves and cranial root of the XI one are attached on the lateral aspect of the brainstem.

169. (c) The superior and inferior colliculi of the midbrain act as visual and auditory reflex centres, respectively.

170. (e) The neurons of the substantia nigra are characterized by the presence of neuromelanin pigments and production of the dopamine.

171. (d) The emergence of trigeminal (V cranial) nerve demarcates its junction with the middle cerebellar peduncle.

172. (d) The motor and main sensory nuclei of the trigeminal nerve, and superior medullary velum are the features exclusively observed in the cross-sections through upper part of the pons.

173. (c) In the lower part of the medulla oblongata, the anterior median fissure is obliterated by the interdigitations of bundles of fibres crossing obliquely, called decussation of the pyramids.

174. (e) The lower medulla is characterized by the pyramidal decussation which leads to the formation of the lateral corticospinal tracts.

175. (d) Each of the superior surface of the cerebellum is supplied by a single superior cerebellar artery, while its inferior surface receives the blood supply from the two (anterior and posterior) inferior cerebellar arteries.

176. (b) The climbing (olivocerebellar) and mossy (spinocerebellar) fibres synapse with its Purkinje cells directly and indirectly (via the granular cells), respectively.

177. (e) The median eminence in the floor of 4th ventricle is marked above the striae medullares by a swelling called facial colliculus.

178. (b) The somatic motor (area 4) and somatic sensory (areas 3,1,2) areas are located in the precentral and postcentral gyri, respectively.

179. (e) The internal capsule is an example of projection fibres.

180. (a) Third ventricle is the narrow median cavity of the diencephalon.

181. (e) The collateral eminence of inferior horn of the lateral ventricle and calcar avis of its posterior horn are produced by the collateral and calcarine sulci, respectively.

182. (c) The limbic system helps in retention of recent memories.

183. (d) Pineal gland and habenula together form the epithalamus.

184. (b) Phylogenetically, the caudate nucleus and putamen of the lentiform nucleus constitute the neostriatum, whereas the globus pallidus forms the paleostriatum.

185. (b) The lateral spinothalamic tract, carrying pain and temperature sensations, is usually involved in the syringomyelia.

186. (b) The pyramidal tract is a two-neuron pathway.

187. (a) Internal capsule is the collection of fibres between lentiform nucleus laterally, and thalamus and the caudate nucleus medially.

188. (b) The optic nerve fibres derived from nasal half of the retina cross at the optic chiasma to enter the opposite optic tract.

189. (b) The ventral and dorsal cochlear nuclei are placed on the corresponding aspects of the inferior cerebellar peduncle.

190. (e) Carotid (Chassaignac's) tubercle is large anterior tubercle of transverse process of 6th cervical vertebra against which the common carotid artery can be effectively compressed.

191. (d) Spinous process of the 7th cervical vertebra is most massive and hence its name, vertebra prominens.

192. (b) The skull is described to be dolicho-, meso- and brachycephalic when the cranial index is less than 75, from 75 to 80 and more than 80, respectively.

193. (e) Osteogenic cells generally bring about complete ossification of sutural ligament but only after the cranial growth ends.

194. (c) The skin of auricle is closely attached with its elastic fibrocartilaginous framework and therefore inflammatory conditions of the auricle are very painful.

195. (d) Fracture of nasal bones usually horizontal and in the lower one-third, is a common occurrence.

196. (b) The lateral margin of orbital opening is formed in its upper and lower halves by frontal and zygomatic bones, respectively.

197. (a) Anterior nasal aperture is piriform in shape.

198. (e) Interior of the orbit is most conveniently approached from lateral side as the eyeball is farthest from its lateral wall.

199. (a) Major contribution (anterior wall, floor and lower part of posterior wall) to the bony external acoustic meatus is derived from tympanic part, while its roof and upper part of posterior wall only are formed by squamous part of temporal bone.

200. (b) Styloid process develops from cartilage (Reichert's) of 2nd pharyngeal (hyoid) arch.

201. (d) Oculomotor, abducent and nasociliary nerves enter the orbit through the tendinous ring.

202. (e) The swelling of scalp produced by cephalohematoma is limited by sutures and therefore corresponds to the shape of the bone.

203. (a) The scalp receives profuse arterial supply from both external carotid (superficial temporal, posterior auricular and occipital branches) as well as internal carotid (supratrochlear and supraorbital branches) arteries.

204. (d) Sympathetic twigs for scalp are derived from superior cervical ganglion.

205. (a) Embryologically, the facial muscles belong to 2nd pharyngeal (hyoid) arch.

206. (b) The investing lamina of cervical fascia extends from mandibular base and superior nuchal line above to pectoral girdle and suprasternal notch below.

207. (c) The floor of the posterior triangle is mainly formed by splenius capitis, levator scapulae and scalenus medius.

208. (b) Cutaneous nerves appearing in posterior triangle are lesser occipital, great auricular, transverse cervical and supraclavicular.

209. (a) External jugular vein is formed at the lower end of parotid gland by the union of posterior division of retromandibular vein and posterior auricular vein.

210. (b) Scalenus anterior is innervated by ventral rami of 4th to 6th cervical nerves.

211. (d) Most of the branches (vertebral, internal thoracic, thyro-cervical and costocervical) spring from the 1st part of subclavian artery while dorsal scapular artery usually arises from its 3rd part.

212. (a) Brachial plexus is formed by the ventral rami of cervical 5, 6, 7 and 8 and thoracic 1 spinal segments.

213. (d) The upper lesion of brachial plexus (Erb-Duchenne or obstetrical paralysis) leads to 'policeman-tip' deformity.

214. (e) The trapezius myocutaneous flap is based on transverse cervical artery and can be used to cover the defects of neck, face and scalp.

215. (c) Thoracolumbar fascia is thin in the thoracic region and continues with its posterior lamina in the lumbar region, below and investing lamina of the deep cervical fascia, above.

216. (a) The boundaries of suboccipital triangle are formed by rectus capitis posterior major and obliquus capitis superior and inferior.

217. (c) Cervical part of facial artery is closely applied to the back of submandibular gland where it arches over posterior belly of digastric and stylohyoid muscle.

218. (b) Facial artery runs anterior to facial vein and traverses a cleft in the modiolus.

219. (e) 'Danger area' of face is a triangular area between angles of mouth and root of nose.

220. (c) The skin of the face derived from the mandibular prominence is supplied by auriculotemporal, buccal and mental branches of mandibular nerve.

221. (d) The medial and lateral parts of the eyelid are drained by submandibular and preauricular lymph nodes, respectively.

222. (d) The preganglionic fibres for lacrimal gland run from superior salivatory nucleus to pterygopalatine ganglion through facial, greater superficial petrosal and nerve of pterygoid canal (Vidian nerve).

223. (e) Lacrimal sac is innervated by infratrochlear nerve.

224. (a) The cranial dura mater consists of an outer endosteal and an inner meningeal layer.

225. (a) Ophthalmic artery and optic nerve run together in the optic canal, while ophthalmic veins traverse through superior orbital fissure.

226. (c) Internal acoustic meatus is traversed by VII and VIII cranial nerves along with labyrinthine artery while IX, X and XI cranial nerves pass through jugular foramen.

227. (a) Internal carotid artery is named as internal because it supplies the structures within the skull.

228. (b) Caroticotympanic and pterygoid branches originate from the petrous part of internal carotid artery.

229. (c) Lesser petrosal nerve carries preganglionic secretomotor fibres from inferior salivatory nucleus to otic ganglion for parotid gland.

230. (d) All the cranial dural venous sinuses ultimately drain into internal jugular vein.

231. (d) Cavernous sinus receives afferents from orbit, vault and cerebrum and drains through superior and inferior petrosal sinuses into sigmoid sinus and internal jugular vein, respectively.

232. (a) The posterior dilated end of superior sagittal sinus is termed as the confluence of sinuses or torcular Herophili.

233. (d) All the striated muscles of orbit except superior oblique and lateral rectus are supplied by oculomotor nerve while the non-striated muscles have sympathetic innervation.

234. (a) The ophthalmic artery, a branch of carotid siphon, enters the optic canal below and lateral to optic nerve.

235. (c) About 8-10 short ciliary nerves emerging from ciliary ganglion carry postganglionic parasympathetic fibres for constrictor pupillae and ciliary muscles, sympathetic fibres for vessels and sensory fibres for eyeball including cornea.

236. (b) Anterior triangle is divided into 4 triangles (muscular, digastric, carotid and corresponding half of the submental) by two bellies of digastric and superior belly of omohyoid.

237. (c) Cervical part of sympathetic chain lies over prevertebral fascia which intervenes between it and anterior vertebral muscles.

238. (d) The lower end of omohyoid is attached to the medial end of the clavicle during foetal life but later in adult life gets attached to the scapula as a result of migration along the clavicle.

239. (a) Masseter, the most superficial muscle of mastication, produces elevation of mandible.

240. (e) Damage of the facial nerve proximal to genicular ganglion leads to total loss of function.

241. (b) The bones contributing to the temporal fossa are parietal, sphenoid, temporal and frontal.

242. (d) Medial aspect of mandibular neck is related to auriculo-temporal nerve, maxillary vein and maxillary artery from above downwards.

243. (b) The main trunk of mandibular nerve is located 4 cm from surface just anterior to mandibular neck.

244. (e) Branches of otic ganglion join the auriculotemporal nerve to supply the parotid gland.

245. (c) Temporomandibular joint is innervated by auriculotemporal and masseteric nerves.

246. (a) Pterygopalatine fossa is bounded by pterygoid process of sphenoid, body of maxilla and perpendicular plate of palatine bone.

247. (c) The anterior and posterior bellies of digastric are derived from 1st and 2nd pharyngeal arches, respectively.

248. (b) The superficial and deep parts of submandibular gland meet behind the posterior border of mylohyoid muscle.

249. (c) The hyoglossus muscle pulls the tongue downwards.

250. (e) The innervation of sublingual gland is derived from lingual nerve, chorda tympani and external carotid sympathetic plexus.

251. (e) Superior thyroid artery is ligated nearer the gland while inferior thyroid artery is tied farther from it to protect the external and recurrent laryngeal nerves, respectively.

252. (c) The cartilaginous tracheal rings are deficient posteriorly for trachealis muscle.

253. (a) The vertebral artery emerges from the 1st part of subclavian artery and ends by meeting its fellow of opposite side at the lower border of pons to form basilar artery .

254. (d) In children, the external carotid artery is smaller than internal carotid artery but in adults both are almost of equal size.

255. (e) The lingual branches of glossopharyngeal nerve receive general and taste sensations from posterior one-third of tongue including sulcus terminalis and vallate papillae.

256. (c) The vagus nerve runs a vertical course behind the groove between internal jugular vein and accompanying carotid artery (internal or common) in the carotid sheath.

257. (b) The spinal root of accessory nerve emerges from anterior grey column of upper 5 cervical spinal segments and ascends between ligamentum denticulatum and dorsal spinal roots.

258. (a) The somatic motor nucleus of hypoglossal nerve is located in the hypoglossal trigone in the lower part of floor of 4th ventricle.

259. (c) The superior, middle and inferior cervical ganglia give somatic branches to anterior primary rami of first four, next two and last two cervical spinal nerves, respectively.

260. (b) The internal jugular vein is represented on the surface by a broad band from ear's lobule to sternal end of clavicle.

261. (a) The cervical plexus is formed by upper 4 cervical ventral rami.

262. (c) Scalenus posterior arises from posterior tubercles of lower cervical vertebral transverse processes and descends to get attached to the 2nd rib.

263. (e) Stellate ganglion block is performed in the region of root of neck to relieve the vascular spasm in the brain and upper limb.

264. (e) All the lymphatics of head and neck ultimately enter the deep cervical lymph nodes whose efferents join to form jugular trunk.

265. (a) Adjacent bodies of lower 6 cervical vertebrae form paired synovial joints near lateral margins and unpaired secondary cartilaginous joints in the centre.

266. (d) The roof of oral cavity proper (hard palate) is innervated by greater palatine and nasopalatine nerves while its floor is supplied by lingual nerve.

267. (b) The buccopharyngeal fascia covers the outer surfaces of the constrictors of pharynx.

268. (c) Fossa of Rosenmuller (pharyngeal recess) is a narrow slit posterior to the opening of Eustachian tube.

269. (d) Posterior one-third of the dorsum of tongue belongs to oropharynx and is innervated by glossopharyngeal nerve for general sensation.

270. (a) Killian's dehiscence is the weakness in the pharyngeal wall in the region of thyropharyngeus below the vocal cords just behind the cricoid lamina.

271. (a) Soft palate is a mobile muscular flap between nasopharynx and oropharynx.

272. (b) The medial two-thirds of the Eustachian tube is cartilaginous while its lateral one-third is osseous.

273. (c) Veins from anterior and posterior halves of the nasal septum drain into facial vein and pterygoid venous plexus, respectively.

274. (d) Only anterior superior quadrant of the lateral wall of the nasal cavity lies in the territory of internal carotid artery while the rest is supplied by external carotid artery.

275. (e) In antrostomy, an artificial opening is made in the inferior meatus to help the drainage of pus from the maxillary sinus.

276. (c) Cricoarytenoid and cricothyroid joints are synovial joints allowing movements of the laryngeal cartilages and thus exerting effects on the vocal cords.

277. (a) Inlet of larynx is directed backwards.

278. (b) Posterior cricoarytenoids are the muscles which open (abduct) the rima glottidis while lateral cricoarytenoid and interarytenoid muscles cause its closure (adduction).

279. (d) The papillae (vallate, fungiform and filiform) are confined to anterior two-thirds of dorsum of tongue.

280. (e) In cases of paralysis of genioglossus, the tongue deviates to the paralysed side during protrusion.

281. (d) To straighten the canal of external acoustic meatus, the auricle is pulled upwards, backwards.

282. (b) The concave lateral surface of the tympanic membrane is directed downwards, laterally and forwards.

283. (d) The upper part of the anterior wall of middle ear has two openings (upper one for tensor tympani and lower one for

Eustachian tube) and the lower part of its anterior wall contains carotid canal.

284. (a) The three ossicles of middle ear, from lateral to medial, are malleus, incus and stapes.

285. (e) The roof of mastoid antrum is formed by tegmen tympani which separates it from middle cranial fossa and temporal lobe.

286. (c) The base of modiolus, which is the axial bony stem for cochlea, lies at the fundus of internal acoustic meatus.

287. (a) The fluid of membranous labyrinth, called endolymph, is separated from the perilymph of scala vestibuli and scala tympani by Reissner's and basilar membranes, respectively.

288. (c) The choroid proper lies internal to the suprachoroid lamina and is composed of three laminae; external vascular, intermediate capillary and internal basal (membrane of Bruch).

289. (b) The lens is a transparent biconvex body with anterior convexity of greater radius than posterior one.

290. (d) Midiguinal point is a point on the inguinal ligament midway between anterior superior iliac spine and pubic symphysis.

291. (a) Addison's plane passes through the tips of 9th costal cartilages and corresponds with the intervertebral disc between lumbar vertebrae 1 and 2.

292. (d) Abdominal viscera lying in its 4 quadrants are liver and gall-bladder in the upper right, stomach and spleen in the upper left, caecum and appendix in the lower right while descending and sigmoid colons in the lower left region.

293. (c) Subcostal (T_{12}) and iliohypogastric (L_1) nerves are muscular as well as cutaneous for the anterior abdominal wall.

294. (b) Caput medusae result from portal hypertension.

295. (b) Below the umbilicus, superficial fascia of anterior abdominal wall is divisible into a superficial fatty layer (of Camper) and a deep membranous layer (of Scarpa).

296. (a) The external oblique muscle of abdomen originates from lower 8 ribs.

297. (d) Plane between internal oblique and transversus abdominis forms neurovascular plane.

298. (c) The costal fibres of transversus abdominis interdigitate with those of diaphragm.

299. (b) Rectus abdominis is inserted over the 5th, 6th and 7th costal cartilages.

300. (a) Rectus sheath is a fibrous compartment with complete anterior wall and incomplete posterior wall.

301. (e) The roof of the inguinal canal is formed by the arched fibres of internal oblique and transversus abdominis.

302. (a) The inguinal canal extends from deep inguinal ring (in fascia tansversalis) to superficial inguinal ring (in aponeurosis of external oblique).

303. (a) The spermatic cord is located partly in the inguinal canal and partly in the scrotum.

304. (d) Anterior one-third of the scrotal skin is supplied by ilioinguinal nerve (L_1) while its posterior two-thirds is innervated by scrotal nerve (S_3).

305. (c) The testis weighs about 10–14 g.

306. (b) Peritoneal fold connecting the stomach with adjacent viscus is called omentum.

307. (b) Greater omentum is also called abdominal police man due to its property of localizing the inflammation.

308. (a) The lesser sac is located behind the stomach and lesser omentum.

309. (e) The lesser and greater curvatures of stomach are directed towards right and left sides, respectively.

310. (c) The capacities of stomach at birth, puberty and adult are about 0.03, 1 and 1.5 litres, respectively.

311. (d) Gastroepiploic arteries are 2 cm from the greater curvature of stomach.

312. (b) The stomach receives its parasympathetic fibres from anterior and posterior vagal trunks which are derived mainly from left and right vagi, respectively.

313. (c) Spleen has inferior, medial (margo intermedialis) and notched superior borders.

314. (d) Majority (85%) show two segments (superior and inferior) while minority (16%) represent three segments (superior, intermediate and inferior) in spleen.

315. (e) Duodenojejunal junction is marked by the attachment of ligament of Treitz.

316. (b) The root of the mesentery extends from the left side of 2nd lumbar vertebra to right sacroiliac joint.

317. (a) 1st and 2nd parts of duodenum lie on the right side of 1st three lumbar vertebrae, 3rd part crosses the 3rd lumbar vertebra while 4th part is related to the left side of 2nd lumbar vertebra.

318. (b) Meckel's diverticulum is persistence of intra-abdominal part of vitellointestinal duct.

319. (c) Prepyloric vein, a surgical guide to pylorus, drains into right gastric vein.

320. (c) Duodenal ulcer commonly involves its anterior wall.

321. (a) The length of pancreas is about 12–15 cm.

322. (e) Cancer of the head of pancreas leads to persisting obstructive jaundice.

323. (e) The width of caecum (7.5 cm) is more than its height (6 cm).

324. (b) Type III (ampullary) caecum is observed in majority (90%) of individuals, while type 1 (infantile), II (quadrate) and IV are present in 2%, 3% and 4% cases, respectively.

325. (a) Mesoappendix is derived from the left leaf of the mesentery.

326. (d) Lymphatics of midgut and hindgut portions of colon drain into superior and inferior mesenteric lymph nodes, respectively.

327. (d) Diverticulosis is the evagination of the mucosa through the wall of intestine.

328. (a) The length of portal vein is approximately 8 cm.

329. (b) The obstruction of portal vein leads to splenomegaly, ascites and varicose veins at the sites of portosystemic anastomoses.

330. (c) The liver is located mainly in the right hypochondriac and epigastric regions of abdomen.

331. (d) Three concavities on posterior aspect of liver are related to (from right to left)—inferior vena cava, vertebral column and oesophagus.

332. (c) The right lobe (physiological) of liver is further divided into anterior, intermediate and posterior segments.

333. (a) The liver receives 80% blood from portal vein while 20% blood from hepatic artery.

334. (c) Cystic artery most commonly arises from right hepatic artery.

335. (b) Common bile duct is about 8 cm in length.

336. (e) The diaphragm helps in respiration, abdominal straining (defaecation, micturition and parturition) and weight lifting.

337. (d) Motor supply of diaphragm is derived from phrenic nerves (C_3–C_5) which are also sensory for its central part whereas sensory supply for its peripheral part is derived from lower intercostal nerves.

338. (e) The quadratus lumborum is covered by anterior and middle layers of thoracolumbar fascia whose posterior layer lies over erector spinae.

339. (c) Iliacus is supplied by femoral nerve while psoas major is innervated directly from ventral rami of upper four lumbar nerves.

340. (e) Genitofemoral nerve descends on the anterior aspect of psoas major while obturator nerve remains medial to it.

341. (a) There are 4 lumbar and 4 sacral sympathetic ganglia on each side but only one ganglion impar in front of coccyx.

342. (c) Lateral paired branches of the abdominal aorta are inferior phrenic, middle suprarenal, renal and gonadal arteries.

343. (b) Paired tributaries of inferior vena cava are common iliac, lumbar and renal veins only while gonadal vein on the right side only joins inferior vena cava while that on left side joins of left renal vein.

344. (c) Right (R) suprarenal is pyramidal (P) while left (L) one is crescentic(C) in shape (Alphabetical order-CLPR).

345. (a) Single suprarenal vein appears from the hilum of each suprarenal gland and drains on the right side into inferior vena cava while on the left side into left renal vein.

346. (d) Perinephric fat intervenes between the capsule of kidney and renal fascia.

347. (e) In case of horseshoe kidney, the pelvis and ureter descend in front of this organ.

348. (b) The ureter descends over psoas major along the line of the tips of lower 4 lumbar transverse processes.

349. (c) The pelvic part of the ureter is supplied by vesical and uterine (in female) arteries.

350. (a) The bony pelvis is divided into true pelvis and false pelvis by the inlet of pelvis.

351. (b) Female pelvis can be divided into 4 types—gynecoid (42%), android (32%), anthropoid (22%) and platypelloid (2%).

352. (e) True conjugate and diagonal conjugate extend from sacral promontory to superior and inferior margins of pubic symphysis, respectively.

353. (b) The piriformis passes through greater sciatic foramen to enter the gluteal region.

354. (c) The tendon of obturator internus gets inserted on the medial aspect of greater trochanter above the trochanteric fossa which itself receives insertion of obturator externus.

355. (e) Coccygeus is well developed and sacrospinous ligament often absent in tailed mammals.

356. (e) In tailed mammals, both pubococcygeus and iliococcygeus components of levator ani get attached to caudal vertebrae only.

357. (c) Visceral pelvic fascia is very thin over distensible viscera but thick and well-defined membrane over non-distensible viscera (e.g. prostatic fascia).

358. (b) The parietal layer of pelvic peritoneum is supplied by a branch from lumbar plexus (obturator nerve).

359. (c) The peritoneum is reflected from anteroinferior surface of uterus to superior surface of urinary bladder directly and anterior vaginal fornix is devoid of peritoneal covering.

360. (b) There are 3 parietal (inferior gluteal, internal pudendal and obturator) and 3 visceral (superior vesical, inferior vesical and middle rectal) branches arising from anterior division of internal iliac artery.

361. (b) Sacral plexus is formed by lumbosacral trunk (L_4, L_5) and ventral rami of upper 4 sacral nerves.

362. (c) The pain is felt when the volume of fluid in the urinary bladder is more than 500 ml.

363. (a) Trigone is a smooth triangular area in the lower part of the interior of the base of urinary bladder.

364. (e) Micturition is a reflex phenomenon occurring at the level of spinal segments S_2–S_4.

365. (b) The length (base to apex) of prostate gland is about 3 cm.

366. (d) Benign prostatic hypertrophy usually involves its mucous and submucous glands while malignancy occurs in main glands of prostate.

367. (e) The lower part of the rectum is named as rectal ampulla.

368. (c) Rectum is drained by superior and middle rectal veins which are tributaries of inferior mesenteric and internal iliac veins, respectively.

369. (e) The anal canal is related anteriorly to perineal body, membranous urethra and bulb of penis in male while perineal body and vagina in female.

370. (e) Lower one-third of anal mucosa is supplied by somatic nerve (inferior rectal branch of pudendal nerve) and therefore is very sensitive.

371. (a) The ovary is located in ovarian fossa bounded anteriorly by obliterated umbilical artery and posteriorly by internal iliac artery and ureter.

372. (c) Ovarian vein is a tributary of inferior vena cava on the right side and left renal vein on the left side.

373. (b) The weight of the uterus is approximately 35g.

374. (c) Three main ligaments supporting the uterus are— pubocervical, Mackenrodt's and uterosacral.

375. (d) The medial two-thirds of fallopian tube is supplied by uterine artery while lateral one-third of the same by ovarian artery.

376. (b) The lengths of anterior and posterior walls of vagina are 7.5 and 9 cm, respectively.

377. (b) The lateral wall of ischiorectal fossa is formed by ischial tuberosity and fascia over obturator internus.

378. (d) Both, pudendal nerve and internal pudendal artery, provide an inferior rectal branch in the posterior part of Alcock's canal.